The Complete Plant-Based Anti-Inflammatory Cookbook 2024

A Beginners Journey to Vegetarian Healing: Delicious Gluten-Free, Whole food Recipes for Soothing Inflammation and Boosting Health. 30-Day Meal Plan Included

Dr Emmy Mack

Copyright © 2024 by Dr Emmy Mack

All rights reserved.

Unauthorized reproduction of any part of this book is strictly prohibited without prior written consent from the publisher or author, except as permitted by applicable copyright law.

This publication aims to offer accurate and authoritative information regarding the subject matter covered. It is sold with the understanding that neither the author nor the publisher is providing legal, investment, accounting, or other professional services. While the author and publisher have made every effort to ensure the accuracy and completeness of the contents of this book, they do not warrant or represent its completeness or accuracy, and disclaim any implied warranties of merchantability or fitness for a particular purpose. No warranty, whether express or implied, is made by the publisher or author regarding the information contained herein.

The advice and strategies presented in this book may not be suitable for your individual situation. It is advisable to seek professional advice when necessary. Neither the publisher nor the author shall be held liable for any loss of profit or any other commercial damages, including but not limited to special, incidental, consequential, personal, or other damages, resulting from the use of the information provided in this book.

CONTENTS

INTRODUCTION 1
    Understanding Inflammation and Diet 2
    Benefits of a Plant-Based Lifestyle 2
    Essential Ingredients for Inflammation Reduction 4

Chapter 1: Breakfast 6
    Blueberry Chia Pudding 6
    Sweet Potato and Black Bean Breakfast Tacos 6
    Quinoa Breakfast Bowl 7
    Turmeric Spiced Oatmeal 8
    Avocado Toast with Pomegranate Seeds 9
    Spinach and Mushroom Breakfast Scramble 10
    Almond Butter Banana Smoothie Bowl 11
    Vegan Breakfast Burrito 11
    Cinnamon Apple Overnight Oats 12
    Green Detox Smoothie 13
    Sweet Potato and Kale Hash 14
    Vegan French Toast 15
    Chia Seed Strawberry Parfait 16
    Pumpkin Spice Muffins 16
    Spelt Flour Pancakes 17

Chapter 2: Beverages 19
    Turmeric Ginger Tea 19
    Green Tea Matcha Latte 19
    Berry Beet Smoothie 20
    Golden Milk Latte 21
    Pineapple Ginger Smoothie 21
    Mint Cucumber Detox Water 22
    Spiced Apple Cider 23
    Anti-Inflammatory Green Juice 24
    Mango Turmeric Smoothie 25
    Hibiscus Iced Tea 25
    Lemon Ginger Infused Water 26
    Pomegranate Green Tea 27
    Cherry Basil Lemonade 27
    Carrot Orange Ginger Juice 28
    Blueberry Basil Smoothie 29

Chapter 3: Soups 30
    Curried Lentil Soup 30

Roasted Tomato Basil Soup 31

Miso Soup with Tofu and Greens 32

Sweet Potato and Carrot Soup... 33

Broccoli and Kale Soup 34

Turmeric Ginger Vegetable Soup 35

Coconut Curry Butternut Squash Soup 36

Spiced Chickpea and Spinach Stew 37

Cauliflower Leek Soup 38

Tomato and Red Pepper Soup 39

Zucchini and Basil Soup 39

Mushroom and Barley Soup... 40

Gingered Carrot Soup 41

Sweet Corn and Quinoa Soup 42

Red Lentil and Spinach Soup 43

Chapter 4: Salads 45

Kale and Avocado Salad 45

Rainbow Quinoa Salad 45

Spinach and Strawberry Salad 46

Roasted Beet and Orange Salad... 47

Cucumber and Tomato Salad with Mint.. 48

Arugula and Pear Salad 49

Warm Lentil and Sweet Potato Salad 49

Broccoli and Cranberry Salad 50

Turmeric Cauliflower Rice Salad 51

Asian Sesame Cabbage Salad 52

Grilled Vegetable Salad.. 53

Mediterranean Farro Salad 54

Mango Black Bean Salad 55

Spicy Thai Peanut Noodle Salad 56

Chapter 5: Main Dishes.. 58

Chickpea and Spinach Patties 58

Black Bean and Sweet Potato Burgers 59

BBQ Jackfruit Sandwiches 60

Vegan Meatloaf with Lentils and Walnuts... 61

Seitan Stir-Fry with Vegetables.. 62

Tempeh Tacos with Avocado 63

Portobello Mushroom Steaks 64

Chickpea and Quinoa Stuffed Peppers 65

Vegan Shepherd's Pie 66

Grilled Tofu with Chimichurri Sauce 67

Eggplant Rollatini with Cashew Ricotta.. 68

- Spicy Lentil and Vegetable Stew ... 69
- Pulled Jackfruit Tacos ... 70
- Vegan Tuna Salad with Chickpeas ... 71
- Watermelon Poke Bowl ... 72

Chapter 6: Snacks & Sides ... 74
- Roasted Chickpeas ... 74
- Baked Sweet Potato Fries ... 75
- Spicy Hummus with Veggie Sticks ... 75
- Avocado Hummus ... 76
- Kale Chips with Nutritional Yeast ... 77
- Stuffed Mini Peppers with Quinoa ... 78
- Garlic and Herb Roasted Nuts ... 79
- Cucumber Avocado Rolls ... 80
- Beetroot Hummus ... 80
- Turmeric Roasted Cauliflower ... 81
- Carrot and Zucchini Fritters ... 82
- Stuffed Mushrooms with Spinach ... 83
- Edamame with Sea Salt ... 84
- Marinated Artichoke Hearts ... 85
- Vegan Cheese Platter ... 85

Chapter 7: Desserts ... 87
- Dark Chocolate Avocado Mousse ... 87
- Coconut Chia Pudding ... 87
- Almond Butter Cookies ... 88
- Baked Cinnamon Apples ... 89
- Berry Chia Parfait ... 90
- Mango Sorbet ... 90
- Matcha Green Tea Ice Cream ... 91
- Vegan Lemon Bars ... 92
- Chocolate-Dipped Strawberries ... 93
- Raw Brownie Bites ... 94
- Pineapple Coconut Smoothie Bowl ... 95
- Pumpkin Pie Bites ... 95

30-DAY MEAL PLAN ... 97
MEASUREMENT CONVERSION TABLE ... 99
CONCLUSION ... 100
RECIPES INDEX ... 101

INTRODUCTION

Welcome to this Plant-Based Anti-Inflammatory Cookbook. With my background as a doctor and dietitian, I have devoted my life to comprehending the significant influence that nutrition has on our well-being. Throughout my experience, I have seen numerous patients who have been dealing with chronic inflammation, facing challenges such as pain, fatigue, and various health issues. From my experience, I've learned that incorporating a diet focused on plants can significantly reduce inflammation and enhance overall well-being.

My journey into the world of plant-based eating began during my medical training. Surrounded by the latest research, I was constantly reminded of the benefits of plant-based diets. However, it was a personal experience that truly opened my eyes. A close family member's diagnosis with an inflammatory condition led us to explore the potential of a plant-based diet. The results were astounding. Their health improved significantly, and a quality of life we thought was lost forever was restored. This profound experience solidified my belief in the power of plant-based eating.

My personal experience, mixed with my professional background, has led me to create this cookbook. I wanted to provide a resource that not only offers delicious and healthy recipes but also educates readers about the science of inflammation and how to combat it with food. Each recipe in this book is meticulously crafted, infused with a personal touch, and most importantly, backed by scientific evidence. They are designed to guide you on a journey towards wellness and vitality.

Regardless of your level of experience with plant-based eating, I hope this cookbook motivates you to appreciate the nourishing benefits of plants. Let's join forces and start our journey towards improved health, savoring every delightful meal along the way.

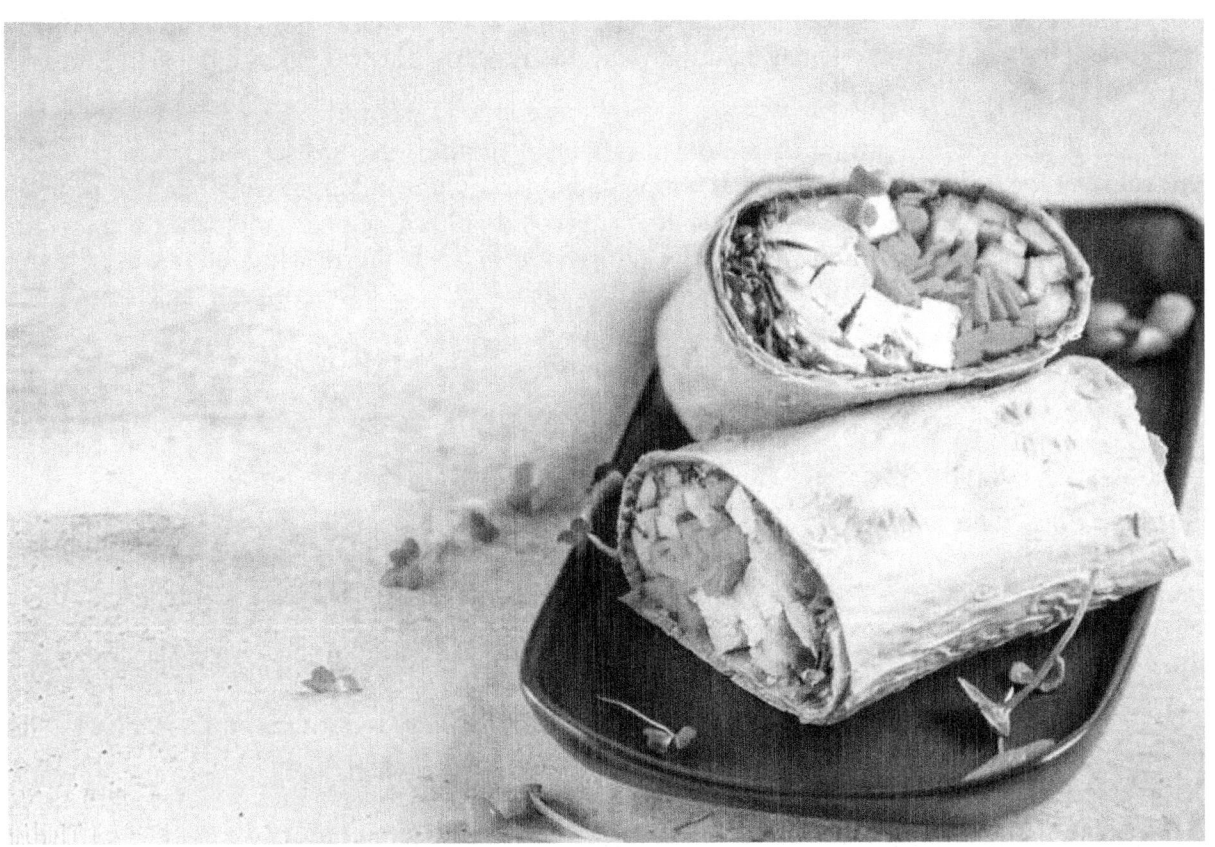

Understanding Inflammation and Diet

Inflammation is a natural response of the immune system that plays a crucial role in healing and safeguarding the body against injury and infection. However, if inflammation persists over time, it can contribute to various health issues such as heart disease, diabetes, arthritis, and certain types of cancer. For the sake of maintaining long-term health, it is important to grasp the significance of diet in managing and preventing chronic inflammation.

Inflammation is a natural biological response to harmful stimuli like pathogens, damaged cells, or irritants. When the body's immune system is activated, it releases chemicals that cause an inflammatory response. This response is often marked by redness, heat, swelling, and pain. This acute inflammation usually doesn't last long and goes away once the healing process is finished. On the other hand, chronic inflammation can last for a long time and lead to continuous harm to tissues and organs.

The role of diet in chronic inflammation is crucial, as it can either worsen or improve the condition. Some foods have the ability to cause inflammation in the body, while others have anti-inflammatory properties that can provide relief and promote healing. Common examples of pro-inflammatory foods are refined sugars, processed foods, trans fats, and red meat. These foods have the potential to cause inflammation in the body, which can contribute to the development and progression of chronic diseases.

In contrast, a diet that focuses on plant-based foods like fruits, vegetables, whole grains, nuts, seeds, and legumes has been proven to have anti-inflammatory effects. These foods contain various beneficial compounds that can help protect the body against oxidative stress and boost its natural defenses. Take spinach and kale, for example. These leafy greens are packed with antioxidants and polyphenols that shield your cells from harm. Berries contain a wealth of vitamins and anti-inflammatory compounds that help to lower inflammation markers. Flaxseeds and walnuts are known for their ability to reduce inflammatory processes.

In addition, some spices and herbs like turmeric, ginger, and garlic have strong anti-inflammatory properties. Extensive research has been conducted on curcumin, the potent compound found in turmeric, due to its remarkable potential in combating inflammation and providing relief from the symptoms of chronic inflammatory conditions.

Adding these foods that reduce inflammation to your diet can significantly impact your overall health and well-being. Opting for a plant-based approach not only helps to reduce inflammation, but also provides your body with vital nutrients that support overall health. This cookbook is filled with mouthwatering recipes that are simple to prepare and promote a healthier, more vibrant life by harnessing the power of plants to combat inflammation.

Benefits of a Plant-Based Lifestyle

Adopting a plant-based lifestyle can bring about a multitude of health benefits, enhancing not only your physical well-being but also your mental and emotional health. From my experience as a doctor and dietitian, I have witnessed the incredible health benefits that come from adopting a plant-based diet. Discover the numerous advantages of embracing a plant-based lifestyle:

1. **Reduces Chronic Inflammation**
   A plant-based diet naturally includes a variety of foods that help reduce inflammation in the body. Include a variety of fruits, vegetables, whole grains, nuts, seeds, and legumes in your diet. These foods are rich in antioxidants, vitamins, minerals, and phytochemicals that can help fight oxidative stress and lower chronic inflammation. Lowering the risk of inflammatory diseases like arthritis, heart disease, and certain cancers is a potential outcome.

2. **Promotes Heart Health**
   Multiple studies have demonstrated the significant reduction in cardiovascular disease risk associated with plant-based diets. Plant-based foods are generally known for their low levels of saturated fats and cholesterol and are rich in fiber and beneficial fats such as omega-3 fatty acids. This combination is beneficial for maintaining healthy blood pressure, reducing LDL cholesterol levels, and promoting overall heart health.
3. **Aids in Weight Management**
   Following a plant-based diet can be a helpful approach for managing weight. Plant-based foods tend to have fewer calories and more fiber than foods that come from animals. This allows you to enjoy bigger servings while reducing calories, making it easier to lose weight and stay healthy. In addition, fiber helps you feel full, which can help you eat fewer calories overall.
4. **Improves Digestive Health**
   Foods rich in fiber, like fruits, vegetables, whole grains, and legumes, help maintain a healthy digestive system by promoting regular bowel movements and supporting a balanced gut microbiome. Having a well-balanced gut microbiome is essential for proper nutrient absorption, a strong immune system, and optimal digestive health.
5. **Enhances Mental Well-Being**
   It is becoming increasingly clear that adopting a diet centered around plants can have a beneficial effect on mental well-being. Plant-based foods rich in nutrients are essential for maintaining brain function and regulating mood. Research has shown that incorporating foods rich in antioxidants and omega-3 fatty acids, like berries and flaxseeds, into your diet may help alleviate symptoms of depression and anxiety.
6. **Supports Sustainable Living**
   Opting for a plant-based lifestyle has numerous advantages for your well-being and the planet. Plant-based diets are more environmentally friendly than animal-based diets, using fewer resources like water and land and producing lower greenhouse gas emissions. Choosing plant-based foods helps promote a sustainable and eco-friendly lifestyle.
7. **Boosts Immune Function**
   Incorporating a variety of fruits, vegetables, nuts, and seeds into your diet is vital for maintaining a robust immune system. Plant foods contain essential nutrients like Vitamins C and E, zinc, and selenium, which play a crucial role in supporting a strong immune system and defending against infections.
8. **Reduces Risk of Chronic Diseases**
   Incorporating a variety of fruits, vegetables, nuts, and seeds into your diet is crucial for maintaining a robust immune system. Plant foods contain essential nutrients like Vitamins C and E, zinc, and selenium, vital to supporting a strong immune system. Research has shown that adopting a plant-based diet can significantly reduce the chances of developing chronic diseases like type 2 diabetes, hypertension, and certain types of cancer. Plant foods contain various beneficial compounds like antioxidants, fiber, and phytonutrients. These compounds help protect against inflammation and oxidative stress, which can contribute to certain health conditions.

Embracing a plant-based lifestyle is a proactive way to improve your overall health and well-being. This cookbook strives to make this transition enjoyable and accessible, offering a range of tasty and healthy recipes that highlight the benefits of plant-based meals. If you're interested in enhancing your well-being, being mindful of the environment, or savoring delicious meals, adopting a plant-based lifestyle can bring many advantages that can significantly improve your life—protecting against infections.

Essential Ingredients for Inflammation Reduction

Adding certain ingredients known for their anti-inflammatory properties to your diet can significantly reduce chronic inflammation and improve your overall health. As a doctor and dietitian, I've discovered certain plant-based ingredients that are highly effective in reducing inflammation. Here's a list of powerful anti-inflammatory foods that you can easily incorporate into your meals:

- **Leafy Greens**
  Spinach, kale, and Swiss chard are rich in vitamins, minerals, and antioxidants, making them healthy choices. These foods also contain a good amount of vitamin K, which has been proven to lower inflammatory markers in the bloodstream.
- **Berries**
  Fruits such as blueberries, strawberries, and raspberries contain antioxidants, specifically anthocyanins, that offer anti-inflammatory benefits. These substances aid in fighting oxidative stress and decreasing inflammation.
- **Nuts and Seeds**
  Almonds, walnuts, flaxseeds, and chia seeds contain nutritious fats, protein, and fiber. These foods have omega-3 fatty acids, which are well-known for their ability to reduce inflammation.
- **Olive Oil**
  Extra virgin olive oil is commonly included in anti-inflammatory diets because of its abundance of monounsaturated fats and antioxidants. One of these antioxidants, oleocanthal, has been found to have similar effects to anti-inflammatory drugs.
- **Turmeric**
  Turmeric contains curcumin, a powerful anti-inflammatory compound. Curcumin can reduce inflammation and is especially effective when consumed with black pepper, which enhances its absorption.
- **Ginger**
  Ginger has potent anti-inflammatory and antioxidant effects. It can help reduce muscle pain, soreness, and chronic inflammation associated with various diseases.
- **Garlic**
  Garlic contains sulfur compounds that stimulate the immune system and reduce inflammation. It is particularly effective in fighting inflammation caused by arthritis.
- **Tomatoes**
  Tomatoes are rich in lycopene, an antioxidant that reduces inflammation and is most effective when cooked. They also provide vitamins C and E, which help reduce inflammatory responses.
- **Whole Grains**
  Whole grains such as brown rice, quinoa, and oats are known for their fiber content, which can help reduce inflammation. They assist in keeping blood sugar levels stable, which helps prevent sudden spikes that can cause inflammation.
- **Legumes**
  Beans, lentils, and other legumes are excellent protein, fiber, and essential nutrient sources. They help reduce inflammation and are a great alternative to animal proteins.
- **Green Tea**
  Green tea contains a high amount of antioxidants, specifically epigallocatechin-3-gallate (EGCG), that have powerful anti-inflammatory properties. Consistently incorporating this into your diet can help lower the chances of developing chronic inflammatory diseases.
- **Cruciferous Vegetables**
  Broccoli, Brussels sprouts, and cauliflower contain sulforaphane, an antioxidant that helps reduce inflammation. It does this by lowering levels of cytokines and nuclear factor kappa B (NF-κB), which are responsible for driving inflammation.
- **Citrus Fruits**

Oranges, lemons, and grapefruits are rich in vitamin C, essential for reducing inflammation. They assist in counteracting free radicals that lead to oxidative stress and inflammation.

- **Avocados**
  Avocados contain a high amount of monounsaturated fats, fiber, and antioxidants. These compounds have the ability to decrease inflammation in both the skin and joints.

Adding these ingredients to your daily meals can assist in managing and reducing chronic inflammation, which can contribute to improved health and well-being. This cookbook provides a clear and straightforward guide to creating mouthwatering, anti-inflammatory meals. It showcases the use of powerful ingredients to enhance your culinary experience.

Chapter 1: Breakfast

Blueberry Chia Pudding

Time to Prepare: 10 minutes
Cooking Time: 0 minutes (refrigeration time: 4 hours or overnight)
Number of Servings: 4

Ingredients:

- 1 cup of unsweetened almond milk
- 1 cup of fresh blueberries (plus extra for topping)
- 1/4 cup of chia seeds
- 1 tablespoon maple syrup
- 1/2 teaspoon of vanilla extract
- 1/2 teaspoon of ground cinnamon

Instructions List:

1. In a blender, combine the almond milk, 1 cup of blueberries, maple syrup, vanilla extract, and ground cinnamon. Blend until smooth.
2. Pour the mixture into a medium-sized bowl and stir in the chia seeds until well mixed.
3. Cover the bowl and refrigerate for at least 4 hours or overnight, allowing the chia seeds to absorb the liquid and thicken.
4. Before serving, stir the pudding to break up any clumps.
5. Divide the chia pudding into 4 servings. Top with additional fresh blueberries before serving.

Nutritional Information (per serving):

- Calories: 120
- Protein: 3g
- Total Fats: 5g
- Fiber: 8g
- Carbohydrates: 18g

Sweet Potato and Black Bean Breakfast Tacos

Time to Prepare: 15 minutes
Cooking Time: 25 minutes
Number of Servings: 4

Ingredients:

- 2 medium sweet potatoes, peeled and diced
- 1 tablespoon olive oil
- 1 teaspoon of ground cumin

- 1 teaspoon of smoked paprika
- Salt and pepper to taste
- 1 can (15 ounces) black beans, drained and rinsed
- 8 small corn tortillas
- 1 avocado, sliced
- 1/4 cup of fresh cilantro, chopped
- 1 lime, cut into wedges
- Hot sauce (optional)

Instructions List:

1. Preheat the oven to 400°F (200°C). Toss the diced sweet potatoes with olive oil, ground cumin, smoked paprika, salt, and pepper. Spread them evenly on a baking sheet.
2. Roast the sweet potatoes in the preheated oven for 20-25 minutes, or until tender and slightly crispy, stirring halfway through.
3. While the sweet potatoes are roasting, heat the black beans in a small saucepan over medium heat until warmed through.
4. Warm the corn tortillas in a dry skillet over medium heat for about 1 minute on each side, or until pliable.
5. To assemble the tacos, divide the roasted sweet potatoes and black beans evenly among the tortillas.
6. Top each taco with avocado slices and fresh cilantro.
7. Serve with lime wedges and hot sauce on the side.

Nutritional Information (per serving):

- Calories: 320
- Protein: 8g
- Total Fats: 11g
- Fiber: 12g
- Carbohydrates: 47g

Quinoa Breakfast Bowl

Time to Prepare: 10 minutes
Cooking Time: 15 minutes
Number of Servings: 4

Ingredients:

- 1 cup of quinoa, rinsed
- 2 cups of water
- 1 cup of fresh berries (strawberries, blueberries, raspberries)
- 1 banana, sliced

- 1/4 cup of almond butter
- 2 tablespoons chia seeds
- 1 tablespoon maple syrup
- 1 teaspoon of ground cinnamon
- 1/4 cup of chopped nuts (almonds, walnuts, or pecans)

Instructions List:

1. In a medium saucepan, bring the quinoa and water to a boil. Reduce heat, cover, and simmer for 15 minutes or until the quinoa is cooked and the water is absorbed. Fluff with a fork.
2. Divide the cooked quinoa into 4 bowls.
3. Top each bowl with fresh berries, banana slices, a dollop of almond butter, chia seeds, a drizzle of maple syrup, ground cinnamon, and chopped nuts.
4. Serve immediately.

Nutritional Information (per serving):

- Calories: 350
- Protein: 10g
- Total Fats: 15g
- Fiber: 10g
- Carbohydrates: 45g

Turmeric Spiced Oatmeal

Time to Prepare: 5 minutes
Cooking Time: 10 minutes
Number of Servings: 4

Ingredients:

- 2 cups of rolled oats
- 4 cups of unsweetened almond milk
- 1 teaspoon of ground turmeric
- 1/2 teaspoon of ground cinnamon
- 1/2 teaspoon of ground ginger
- 1 tablespoon maple syrup
- 1/4 cup of chopped walnuts
- 1/4 cup of raisins
- Fresh berries for topping (optional)

Instructions List:

1. In a medium saucepan, combine the rolled oats and almond milk. Bring to a boil over medium heat.

2. Reduce heat and stir in ground turmeric, ground cinnamon, and ground ginger. Simmer for about 5-7 minutes, stirring occasionally, until the oats are creamy.
3. Stir in the maple syrup, chopped walnuts, and raisins.
4. Divide the oatmeal into 4 bowls. Top with fresh berries if desired.
5. Serve immediately.

Nutritional Information (per serving):

- Calories: 300
- Protein: 7g
- Total Fats: 10g
- Fiber: 7g
- Carbohydrates: 45g

Avocado Toast with Pomegranate Seeds

Time to Prepare: 10 minutes
Cooking Time: 0 minutes
Number of Servings: 4

Ingredients:

- 4 slices whole grain bread
- 2 ripe avocados
- 1/2 cup of pomegranate seeds
- 1 tablespoon lemon juice
- Salt and pepper to taste
- 1/4 teaspoon of red pepper flakes (optional)

Instructions List:

1. Toast the slices of whole grain bread until golden brown.
2. In a bowl, mash the avocados with lemon juice, salt, and pepper.
3. Spread the mashed avocado evenly on each slice of toasted bread.
4. Sprinkle pomegranate seeds and red pepper flakes (if using) over the avocado.
5. Serve immediately.

Nutritional Information (per serving):

- Calories: 280
- Protein: 6g
- Total Fats: 18g
- Fiber: 9g
- Carbohydrates: 26g

Spinach and Mushroom Breakfast Scramble

Time to Prepare: 10 minutes
Cooking Time: 10 minutes
Number of Servings: 4

Ingredients:

- 1 tablespoon olive oil
- 1 small onion, chopped
- 2 cloves garlic, minced
- 1 cup of mushrooms, sliced
- 1 block (14 ounces) firm tofu, crumbled
- 1 teaspoon of ground turmeric
- 1/2 teaspoon of ground cumin
- Salt and pepper to taste
- 4 cups of fresh spinach, roughly chopped
- 1/4 cup of nutritional yeast
- 2 tablespoons fresh parsley, chopped

Instructions List:

1. In a large skillet, heat the olive oil over medium heat. Add the onion and garlic, and sauté until fragrant and translucent, about 3 minutes.
2. Add the mushrooms and cook until they release their moisture and begin to brown, about 5 minutes.
3. Add the crumbled tofu, ground turmeric, ground cumin, salt, and pepper. Stir well to combine and cook for another 2-3 minutes.
4. Add the chopped spinach and cook until wilted, about 2 minutes.
5. Stir in the nutritional yeast and fresh parsley. Mix well and cook for another minute.
6. Serve immediately.

Nutritional Information (per serving):

- Calories: 180
- Protein: 14g
- Total Fats: 9g
- Fiber: 5g
- Carbohydrates: 12g

Almond Butter Banana Smoothie Bowl

Time to Prepare: 10 minutes
Cooking Time: 0 minutes
Number of Servings: 2

Ingredients:

- 2 frozen bananas, sliced
- 1/2 cup of unsweetened almond milk
- 2 tablespoons almond butter
- 1 tablespoon chia seeds
- 1/2 teaspoon of ground cinnamon
- 1/4 cup of granola (optional)
- Fresh berries for topping
- Sliced almonds for topping

Instructions List:

1. In a blender, combine the frozen bananas, almond milk, almond butter, chia seeds, and ground cinnamon. Blend until smooth and creamy.
2. Divide the smoothie mixture into two bowls.
3. Top with granola, fresh berries, and sliced almonds.
4. Serve immediately.

Nutritional Information (per serving):

- Calories: 320
- Protein: 7g
- Total Fats: 15g
- Fiber: 8g
- Carbohydrates: 42g

Vegan Breakfast Burrito

Time to Prepare: 15 minutes
Cooking Time: 15 minutes
Number of Servings: 4

Ingredients:

- 1 tablespoon olive oil
- 1 small onion, chopped
- 2 cloves garlic, minced
- 1 red bell pepper, chopped

- 1 can (15 ounces) black beans, drained and rinsed
- 1 teaspoon of ground cumin
- 1/2 teaspoon of smoked paprika
- Salt and pepper to taste
- 1 block (14 ounces) firm tofu, crumbled
- 4 large whole grain tortillas
- 1 avocado, sliced
- 1/4 cup of salsa
- 2 tablespoons fresh cilantro, chopped

Instructions List:

1. In a large skillet, heat the olive oil over medium heat. Add the onion and garlic, and sauté until fragrant and translucent, about 3 minutes.
2. Add the red bell pepper and cook until softened, about 5 minutes.
3. Stir in the black beans, ground cumin, smoked paprika, salt, and pepper. Cook for another 2-3 minutes.
4. Add the crumbled tofu to the skillet, mixing well with the vegetables and beans. Cook for another 5 minutes, stirring occasionally.
5. Warm the tortillas in a dry skillet or microwave until pliable.
6. Divide the tofu mixture evenly among the tortillas. Top each with avocado slices, salsa, and fresh cilantro.
7. Roll up the tortillas to form burritos. Serve immediately.

Nutritional Information (per serving):

- Calories: 350
- Protein: 14g
- Total Fats: 15g
- Fiber: 12g
- Carbohydrates: 40g

Cinnamon Apple Overnight Oats

Time to Prepare: 10 minutes
Cooking Time: 0 minutes (refrigeration time: overnight)
Number of Servings: 4

Ingredients:

- 2 cups of rolled oats
- 2 cups of unsweetened almond milk
- 1 cup of unsweetened applesauce
- 1 apple, diced

- 2 tablespoons chia seeds
- 1 tablespoon maple syrup
- 1 teaspoon of ground cinnamon
- 1/2 teaspoon of vanilla extract
- 1/4 cup of chopped walnuts

Instructions List:

1. In a large bowl, combine the rolled oats, almond milk, applesauce, diced apple, chia seeds, maple syrup, ground cinnamon, and vanilla extract. Mix well.
2. Divide the mixture evenly into 4 jars or containers.
3. Top each serving with chopped walnuts.
4. Cover and refrigerate overnight.
5. Serve chilled.

Nutritional Information (per serving):

- Calories: 290
- Protein: 6g
- Total Fats: 10g
- Fiber: 7g
- Carbohydrates: 42g

Green Detox Smoothie

Time to Prepare: 5 minutes
Cooking Time: 0 minutes
Number of Servings: 2

Ingredients:

- 2 cups of fresh spinach
- 1 cup of unsweetened almond milk
- 1 banana, frozen
- 1 apple, cored and chopped
- 1/2 avocado
- 1 tablespoon chia seeds
- 1 tablespoon fresh lemon juice
- 1/2 teaspoon of ground ginger

Instructions List:

1. In a blender, combine the spinach, almond milk, frozen banana, apple, avocado, chia seeds, lemon juice, and ground ginger.

2. Blend until smooth.
3. Pour into two glasses and serve immediately.

Nutritional Information (per serving):

- Calories: 220
- Protein: 4g
- Total Fats: 11g
- Fiber: 9g
- Carbohydrates: 30g

Sweet Potato and Kale Hash

Time to Prepare: 10 minutes
Cooking Time: 20 minutes
Number of Servings: 4

Ingredients:

- 2 tablespoons olive oil
- 1 large onion, chopped
- 2 cloves garlic, minced
- 2 large sweet potatoes, peeled and diced
- 1 teaspoon of ground cumin
- 1/2 teaspoon of smoked paprika
- Salt and pepper to taste
- 4 cups of kale, stems removed and chopped
- 1/4 cup of fresh parsley, chopped

Instructions List:

1. In a large skillet, heat the olive oil over medium heat. Add the onion and garlic, and sauté until fragrant and translucent, about 3 minutes.
2. Add the diced sweet potatoes, ground cumin, smoked paprika, salt, and pepper. Cook, stirring occasionally, until the sweet potatoes are tender and slightly crispy, about 15 minutes.
3. Add the chopped kale to the skillet and cook until wilted, about 2-3 minutes.
4. Stir in the fresh parsley.
5. Serve immediately.

Nutritional Information (per serving):

- Calories: 200
- Protein: 4g
- Total Fats: 9g

- Fiber: 5g
- Carbohydrates: 29g

Vegan French Toast

Time to Prepare: 10 minutes
Cooking Time: 10 minutes
Number of Servings: 4

Ingredients:

- 1 cup of unsweetened almond milk
- 1 tablespoon ground flaxseed
- 1 tablespoon nutritional yeast
- 1 teaspoon of ground cinnamon
- 1/2 teaspoon of ground nutmeg
- 1 teaspoon of vanilla extract
- 8 slices whole grain bread
- 2 tablespoons coconut oil
- Fresh berries for topping (optional)
- Maple syrup for serving

Instructions List:

1. In a shallow bowl, whisk together the almond milk, ground flaxseed, nutritional yeast, ground cinnamon, ground nutmeg, and vanilla extract. Let the mixture sit for 5 minutes to thicken.
2. Heat a large skillet over medium heat and add 1 tablespoon of coconut oil.
3. Dip each slice of bread into the almond milk mixture, ensuring both sides are well-coated.
4. Place the coated bread slices in the skillet and cook until golden brown, about 3-4 minutes on each side.
5. Repeat with the remaining bread slices, adding more coconut oil to the skillet as needed.
6. Serve the French toast topped with fresh berries and a drizzle of maple syrup.

Nutritional Information (per serving):

- Calories: 300
- Protein: 8g
- Total Fats: 12g
- Fiber: 6g
- Carbohydrates: 40g

Chia Seed Strawberry Parfait

Time to Prepare: 10 minutes
Cooking Time: 0 minutes (refrigeration time: 2 hours)
Number of Servings: 2

Ingredients:

- 1 cup of unsweetened almond milk
- 1/4 cup of chia seeds
- 1 tablespoon maple syrup
- 1 teaspoon of vanilla extract
- 1 cup of fresh strawberries, sliced
- 1/2 cup of granola (optional)
- Fresh mint leaves for garnish (optional)

Instructions List:

1. In a bowl, whisk together the almond milk, chia seeds, maple syrup, and vanilla extract.
2. Cover the bowl and refrigerate for at least 2 hours, or overnight, until the chia pudding thickens.
3. Once the chia pudding is set, layer it in serving glasses or jars with sliced strawberries and granola.
4. Repeat the layers until the glasses are filled.
5. Garnish with fresh mint leaves, if desired.
6. Serve chilled.

Nutritional Information (per serving):

- Calories: 250
- Protein: 6g
- Total Fats: 10g
- Fiber: 10g
- Carbohydrates: 35g

Pumpkin Spice Muffins

Time to Prepare: 15 minutes
Cooking Time: 20 minutes
Number of Servings: 12

Ingredients:

- 2 cups of whole wheat flour
- 1/2 cup of coconut sugar
- 1 tablespoon baking powder
- 1 teaspoon of ground cinnamon

- 1/2 teaspoon of ground nutmeg
- 1/4 teaspoon of ground cloves
- 1/4 teaspoon of ground ginger
- 1/2 teaspoon of salt
- 1 cup of unsweetened almond milk
- 1 cup of canned pumpkin puree
- 1/4 cup of coconut oil, melted
- 1 teaspoon of vanilla extract

Instructions List:

1. Preheat the oven to 375°F (190°C). Line a muffin tin with paper liners or grease with coconut oil.
2. In a large bowl, whisk together the whole wheat flour, coconut sugar, baking powder, ground cinnamon, ground nutmeg, ground cloves, ground ginger, and salt.
3. In a separate bowl, combine the almond milk, pumpkin puree, melted coconut oil, and vanilla extract.
4. Pour the wet ingredients into the dry ingredients and stir until just mixed. Be careful not to overmix.
5. Divide the batter evenly among the muffin cups, filling each about 2/3 full.
6. Bake for 18-20 minutes, or until a toothpick inserted into the center of a muffin comes out clean.
7. Allow the muffins to cool in the tin for 5 minutes, then transfer to a wire rack to cool completely.

Nutritional Information (per serving):

- Calories: 160
- Protein: 3g
- Total Fats: 6g
- Fiber: 3g
- Carbohydrates: 25g

Spelt Flour Pancakes

Time to Prepare: 10 minutes
Cooking Time: 15 minutes
Number of Servings: 4 (approximately 12 pancakes)

Ingredients:

- 2 cups of spelt flour
- 2 tablespoons coconut sugar
- 1 tablespoon baking powder
- 1/2 teaspoon of salt
- 2 cups of unsweetened almond milk

- 2 tablespoons coconut oil, melted
- 1 teaspoon of vanilla extract

Instructions List:

1. In a large mixing bowl, whisk together the spelt flour, coconut sugar, baking powder, and salt.
2. In a separate bowl, mix the almond milk, melted coconut oil, and vanilla extract.
3. Pour the wet ingredients into the dry ingredients and stir until just mixed. Be careful not to overmix; a few lumps are okay.
4. Heat a non-stick skillet or griddle over medium heat and lightly grease with coconut oil or cooking spray.
5. Pour about 1/4 cup of batter onto the skillet for each pancake.
6. Cook until bubbles form on the surface of the pancake, then flip and cook until golden brown on the other side, about 2-3 minutes per side.
7. Repeat with the remaining batter, greasing the skillet as needed.
8. Serve warm with your favorite toppings such as fresh fruit, maple syrup, or nut butter.

Nutritional Information (per serving, approximately 3 pancakes):

- Calories: 300
- Protein: 7g
- Total Fats: 10g
- Fiber: 5g
- Carbohydrates: 45g

Chapter 2: Beverages

Turmeric Ginger Tea

Time to Prepare: 5 minutes
Cooking Time: 10 minutes
Number of Servings: 2

Ingredients:

- 2 cups of water
- 1 teaspoon of ground turmeric
- 1 teaspoon of grated ginger
- 1 cinnamon stick
- 1 tablespoon maple syrup or agave syrup (optional)
- Juice of 1/2 lemon (optional)

Instructions List:

1. In a small saucepan, bring the water to a boil.
2. Add the ground turmeric, grated ginger, and cinnamon stick to the boiling water.
3. Reduce the heat and let the mixture simmer for about 10 minutes.
4. Strain the tea into mugs using a fine mesh strainer.
5. Stir in maple syrup or agave syrup and lemon juice, if using.
6. Serve hot.

Nutritional Information (per serving):

- Calories: 15
- Protein: 0g
- Total Fats: 0g
- Fiber: 0g
- Carbohydrates: 4g

Green Tea Matcha Latte

Time to Prepare: 5 minutes
Cooking Time: 5 minutes
Number of Servings: 1

Ingredients:

- 1 teaspoon of matcha green tea powder
- 1 cup of unsweetened almond milk or oat milk
- 1 teaspoon of maple syrup or agave syrup (optional)

- Hot water (about 1/4 cup of)

Instructions List:

1. In a small bowl, whisk the matcha green tea powder with a small amount of hot water to create a smooth paste.
2. Heat the almond milk or oat milk in a small saucepan over medium heat until hot but not boiling.
3. Pour the hot milk into a mug.
4. Add the matcha paste to the mug with the hot milk.
5. Stir well until the matcha paste is fully dissolved into the milk.
6. If desired, sweeten with maple syrup or agave syrup.
7. Enjoy hot.

Nutritional Information (per serving):

- Calories: 40
- Protein: 2g
- Total Fats: 2g
- Fiber: 1g
- Carbohydrates: 4g

Berry Beet Smoothie

Time to Prepare: 5 minutes
Cooking Time: 0 minutes
Number of Servings: 2

Ingredients:

- 1 cup of frozen mixed berries (such as strawberries, blueberries, raspberries)
- 1 small beet, peeled and diced
- 1 ripe banana
- 1 cup of unsweetened almond milk or coconut water
- 1 tablespoon chia seeds
- 1 tablespoon hemp seeds
- 1 tablespoon maple syrup or agave syrup (optional)

Instructions List:

1. Place all ingredients in a blender.
2. Blend until smooth and creamy.
3. Taste and adjust sweetness if desired by adding maple syrup or agave syrup.
4. Pour into glasses and serve immediately.

Nutritional Information (per serving):

- Calories: 180
- Protein: 5g
- Total Fats: 6g
- Fiber: 8g
- Carbohydrates: 30g

Golden Milk Latte

Time to Prepare: 5 minutes
Cooking Time: 5 minutes
Number of Servings: 1

Ingredients:

- 1 cup of unsweetened almond milk or coconut milk
- 1 teaspoon of ground turmeric
- 1/2 teaspoon of ground cinnamon
- 1/4 teaspoon of ground ginger
- 1 tablespoon maple syrup or agave syrup (optional)
- Pinch of ground black pepper

Instructions List:

1. In a small saucepan, heat the almond milk or coconut milk over medium heat until hot but not boiling.
2. Whisk in the ground turmeric, ground cinnamon, ground ginger, and maple syrup or agave syrup.
3. Continue to heat the mixture for 2-3 minutes, stirring occasionally, until fragrant.
4. Remove from heat and pour the golden milk into a mug.
5. Sprinkle a pinch of ground black pepper on top.
6. Stir well before serving.

Nutritional Information (per serving):

- Calories: 60
- Protein: 1g
- Total Fats: 2g
- Fiber: 1g
- Carbohydrates: 10g

Pineapple Ginger Smoothie

Time to Prepare: 5 minutes
Cooking Time: 0 minutes
Number of Servings: 2

Ingredients:

- 2 cups of fresh pineapple chunks
- 1 banana
- 1-inch piece of fresh ginger, peeled and grated
- 1 cup of unsweetened coconut water or almond milk
- 1 tablespoon chia seeds
- Ice cubes (optional)

Instructions List:

1. Place all ingredients in a blender.
2. Blend until smooth and creamy.
3. If desired, add ice cubes for a colder consistency and blend again.
4. Pour into glasses and serve immediately.

Nutritional Information (per serving):

- Calories: 120
- Protein: 3g
- Total Fats: 2g
- Fiber: 6g
- Carbohydrates: 26g

Mint Cucumber Detox Water

Time to Prepare: 5 minutes
Cooking Time: 0 minutes
Number of Servings: 4

Ingredients:

- 1 cucumber, thinly sliced
- 1 lemon, thinly sliced
- 10-12 fresh mint leaves
- 4 cups of filtered water
- Ice cubes (optional)

Instructions List:

1. In a large pitcher, combine the cucumber slices, lemon slices, and fresh mint leaves.
2. Pour the filtered water over the ingredients in the pitcher.
3. Stir gently to mix the ingredients.
4. Cover the pitcher and refrigerate for at least 1 hour to allow the flavors to infuse.

5. Serve chilled, adding ice cubes if desired.

Nutritional Information (per serving):

- Calories: 0
- Protein: 0g
- Total Fats: 0g
- Fiber: 0g
- Carbohydrates: 0g

Spiced Apple Cider

Time to Prepare: 5 minutes
Cooking Time: 30 minutes
Number of Servings: 4

Ingredients:

- 4 cups of apple juice (unsweetened)
- 2 cinnamon sticks
- 4 whole cloves
- 1/2 teaspoon of ground nutmeg
- 1/2 teaspoon of ground ginger
- 1/4 teaspoon of ground allspice
- 1/4 teaspoon of ground cardamom
- 1 tablespoon maple syrup or agave syrup (optional)
- Slices of apple and/or orange for garnish (optional)

Instructions List:

1. In a large pot, combine the apple juice, cinnamon sticks, whole cloves, ground nutmeg, ground ginger, ground allspice, and ground cardamom.
2. Bring the mixture to a boil over medium-high heat.
3. Once boiling, reduce the heat to low and let the cider simmer for about 30 minutes, stirring occasionally.
4. Remove the pot from heat and let the cider cool slightly.
5. Strain the cider through a fine mesh strainer to remove the spices.
6. If desired, stir in maple syrup or agave syrup for added sweetness.
7. Serve the spiced apple cider warm.
8. Garnish each serving with slices of apple and/or orange, if desired.

Nutritional Information (per serving):

- Calories: 120
- Protein: 0g

- Total Fats: 0g
- Fiber: 0g
- Carbohydrates: 30g

Anti-Inflammatory Green Juice

Time to Prepare: 10 minutes
Cooking Time: 0 minutes
Number of Servings: 2

Ingredients:

- 2 large handfuls of spinach
- 1 cucumber
- 2 stalks of celery
- 1 green apple
- 1 inch piece of ginger
- 1 lemon, peeled
- 1 tablespoon fresh parsley
- 1 tablespoon fresh cilantro
- 1 cup of filtered water
- Ice cubes (optional)

Instructions List:

1. Wash all the fruits and vegetables thoroughly.
2. Cut the cucumber, celery, and green apple into chunks that will fit into your juicer.
3. Peel the lemon and ginger.
4. Add all ingredients to a juicer, alternating between the leafy greens and harder produce for easier juicing.
5. Juice until all ingredients are processed.
6. If desired, strain the juice through a fine mesh strainer or cheesecloth to remove excess pulp.
7. Serve the green juice immediately over ice cubes if desired.

Nutritional Information (per serving):

- Calories: 70
- Protein: 2g
- Total Fats: 1g
- Fiber: 5g
- Carbohydrates: 18g

Mango Turmeric Smoothie

Time to Prepare: 5 minutes
Cooking Time: 0 minutes
Number of Servings: 2

Ingredients:

- 1 cup of frozen mango chunks
- 1 ripe banana
- 1 cup of unsweetened almond milk
- 1/2 teaspoon of ground turmeric
- 1/2 teaspoon of ground cinnamon
- 1 tablespoon chia seeds
- 1 tablespoon hemp seeds
- Ice cubes (optional)

Instructions List:

1. In a blender, combine the frozen mango chunks, ripe banana, almond milk, ground turmeric, ground cinnamon, chia seeds, and hemp seeds.
2. Blend on high speed until smooth and creamy.
3. If desired, add ice cubes to achieve a colder consistency and blend again.
4. Pour the smoothie into glasses and serve immediately.

Nutritional Information (per serving):

- Calories: 200
- Protein: 6g
- Total Fats: 8g
- Fiber: 8g
- Carbohydrates: 30g

Hibiscus Iced Tea

Time to Prepare: 5 minutes
Cooking Time: 10 minutes
Number of Servings: 4

Ingredients:

- 4 cups of water
- 4 tablespoons dried hibiscus flowers
- 2 tablespoons maple syrup or agave syrup (optional)
- Slices of orange or lemon for garnish (optional)

- Fresh mint leaves for garnish (optional)
- Ice cubes

Instructions List:

1. In a medium saucepan, bring the water to a boil.
2. Add the dried hibiscus flowers to the boiling water.
3. Reduce the heat to low and let the hibiscus steep for about 10 minutes.
4. Remove the saucepan from heat and strain the hibiscus tea into a pitcher.
5. Stir in maple syrup or agave syrup if desired, adjusting sweetness to taste.
6. Allow the tea to cool to room temperature, then refrigerate until chilled.
7. Serve the hibiscus iced tea over ice cubes, garnished with slices of orange or lemon and fresh mint leaves if desired.

Nutritional Information (per serving):

- Calories: 10
- Protein: 0g
- Total Fats: 0g
- Fiber: 0g
- Carbohydrates: 3g

Lemon Ginger Infused Water

Time to Prepare: 5 minutes
Cooking Time: 0 minutes
Number of Servings: 4

Ingredients:

- 4 cups of water
- 1 lemon, thinly sliced
- 1-inch piece of fresh ginger, thinly sliced

Instructions List:

1. In a pitcher, combine the water, lemon slices, and ginger slices.
2. Stir gently to mix the ingredients.
3. Cover the pitcher and refrigerate for at least 1 hour to allow the flavors to infuse.
4. Serve the infused water chilled, either over ice cubes or as is.

Nutritional Information (per serving):

- Calories: 0
- Protein: 0g
- Total Fats: 0g

- Fiber: 0g
- Carbohydrates: 0g

Pomegranate Green Tea

Time to Prepare: 5 minutes
Cooking Time: 5 minutes
Number of Servings: 2

Ingredients:

- 2 cups of water
- 2 green tea bags
- 1/2 cup of pomegranate juice (unsweetened)
- 1 tablespoon maple syrup or agave syrup (optional)
- Slices of lemon for garnish (optional)
- Ice cubes

Instructions List:

1. In a small saucepan, bring the water to a boil.
2. Remove the saucepan from heat and add the green tea bags.
3. Let the tea steep for about 3-5 minutes, depending on desired strength.
4. Remove the tea bags and discard.
5. Stir in the pomegranate juice and maple syrup or agave syrup if desired.
6. Allow the tea to cool to room temperature, then refrigerate until chilled.
7. Serve the pomegranate green tea over ice cubes, garnished with slices of lemon if desired.

Nutritional Information (per serving):

- Calories: 40
- Protein: 0g
- Total Fats: 0g
- Fiber: 0g
- Carbohydrates: 10g

Cherry Basil Lemonade

Time to Prepare: 10 minutes
Cooking Time: 0 minutes
Number of Servings: 4

Ingredients:

- 1 cup of fresh cherries, pitted

- 1/4 cup of fresh basil leaves
- 1/2 cup of freshly squeezed lemon juice
- 4 cups of water
- 2 tablespoons maple syrup or agave syrup (optional)
- Ice cubes
- Fresh basil leaves and cherry slices for garnish (optional)

Instructions List:

1. In a blender, combine the pitted cherries, basil leaves, lemon juice, water, and maple syrup or agave syrup.
2. Blend on high speed until smooth.
3. Strain the mixture through a fine mesh strainer into a pitcher to remove any pulp.
4. Taste and adjust sweetness by adding more maple syrup or agave syrup if desired.
5. Refrigerate the cherry basil lemonade until chilled.
6. Serve over ice cubes, garnished with fresh basil leaves and cherry slices if desired.

Nutritional Information (per serving):

- Calories: 40
- Protein: 1g
- Total Fats: 0g
- Fiber: 1g
- Carbohydrates: 10g

Carrot Orange Ginger Juice

Time to Prepare: 10 minutes
Cooking Time: 0 minutes
Number of Servings: 2

Ingredients:

- 4 large carrots, peeled and chopped
- 2 oranges, peeled and segmented
- 1-inch piece of fresh ginger, peeled
- 1/2 cup of water
- Ice cubes (optional)

Instructions List:

1. In a juicer, juice the carrots, oranges, and ginger.
2. If desired, dilute the juice with water for a milder flavor.
3. Stir well to combine.

4. Serve the carrot orange ginger juice over ice cubes if desired.

Nutritional Information (per serving):

- Calories: 80
- Protein: 2g
- Total Fats: 0g
- Fiber: 5g
- Carbohydrates: 20g

Blueberry Basil Smoothie

Time to Prepare: 5 minutes
Cooking Time: 0 minutes
Number of Servings: 2

Ingredients:

- 2 cups of fresh or frozen blueberries
- 1 ripe banana
- 1/4 cup of fresh basil leaves
- 1 cup of unsweetened almond milk
- 1 tablespoon chia seeds
- 1 tablespoon hemp seeds
- Ice cubes (optional)

Instructions List:

1. In a blender, combine the blueberries, banana, basil leaves, almond milk, chia seeds, and hemp seeds.
2. Blend on high speed until smooth and creamy.
3. If desired, add ice cubes for a colder consistency and blend again.
4. Pour the smoothie into glasses and serve immediately.

Nutritional Information (per serving):

- Calories: 160
- Protein: 4g
- Total Fats: 6g
- Fiber: 8g
- Carbohydrates: 25g

Chapter 3: Soups

Curried Lentil Soup

Time to Prepare: 10 minutes
Cooking Time: 30 minutes
Number of Servings: 4

Ingredients:

- 1 tablespoon olive oil
- 1 onion, diced
- 2 cloves garlic, minced
- 2 carrots, diced
- 2 celery stalks, diced
- 1 tablespoon curry powder
- 1 teaspoon of ground turmeric
- 1 teaspoon of ground cumin
- 1 cup of dried green lentils, rinsed and drained
- 4 cups of vegetable broth
- 1 (14 oz) can diced tomatoes
- Salt and pepper to taste
- Fresh cilantro for garnish (optional)

Instructions List:

1. Heat the olive oil in a large pot over medium heat.
2. Add the diced onion and cook until softened, about 5 minutes.
3. Add the minced garlic, diced carrots, and diced celery to the pot. Cook for another 5 minutes, stirring occasionally.
4. Stir in the curry powder, ground turmeric, and ground cumin, and cook for 1 minute until fragrant.
5. Add the rinsed lentils, vegetable broth, and diced tomatoes to the pot. Stir well to combine.
6. Bring the soup to a boil, then reduce the heat to low and let it simmer for about 20-25 minutes, or until the lentils are tender.
7. Season the soup with salt and pepper to taste.
8. Serve the curried lentil soup hot, garnished with fresh cilantro if desired.

Nutritional Information (per serving):

- Calories: 250
- Protein: 12g
- Total Fats: 4g

- Fiber: 10g
- Carbohydrates: 40g

Roasted Tomato Basil Soup

Time to Prepare: 10 minutes
Cooking Time: 40 minutes
Number of Servings: 4

Ingredients:

- 1 kg tomatoes, halved
- 2 tablespoons olive oil
- 1 onion, chopped
- 3 cloves garlic, minced
- 1 tablespoon tomato paste
- 4 cups of vegetable broth
- 1/4 cup of fresh basil leaves
- Salt and pepper to taste

Instructions List:

1. Preheat the oven to 200°C (400°F).
2. Place the halved tomatoes on a baking sheet, drizzle with olive oil, and season with salt and pepper.
3. Roast the tomatoes in the preheated oven for 25-30 minutes, or until they are softened and caramelized.
4. In a large pot, heat the remaining olive oil over medium heat. Add the chopped onion and cook until softened, about 5 minutes.
5. Add the minced garlic to the pot and cook for another minute until fragrant.
6. Stir in the tomato paste and cook for 2-3 minutes to enhance its flavor.
7. Add the roasted tomatoes (including any juices from the baking sheet) to the pot, along with the vegetable broth.
8. Bring the soup to a simmer and let it cook for 10-15 minutes to allow the flavors to meld together.
9. Use an immersion blender to blend the soup until smooth.
10. Stir in the fresh basil leaves and season the soup with salt and pepper to taste.
11. Serve the roasted tomato basil soup hot.

Nutritional Information (per serving):

- Calories: 180
- Protein: 4g
- Total Fats: 10g
- Fiber: 5g

- Carbohydrates: 20g

Miso Soup with Tofu and Greens

Time to Prepare: 10 minutes
Cooking Time: 10 minutes
Number of Servings: 4

Ingredients:

- 4 cups of vegetable broth
- 3 tablespoons white miso paste
- 1 block (about 200g) firm tofu, diced
- 2 cups of chopped greens (such as spinach, kale, or bok choy)
- 2 green onions, thinly sliced
- 1 tablespoon soy sauce or tamari
- 1 tablespoon rice vinegar
- 1 tablespoon sesame oil
- 1 teaspoon of grated ginger
- 2 cloves garlic, minced
- Red pepper flakes (optional)
- Fresh cilantro or parsley for garnish (optional)

Instructions List:

1. In a large pot, bring the vegetable broth to a simmer over medium heat.
2. In a small bowl, whisk together the white miso paste with a ladleful of hot broth until smooth.
3. Add the miso mixture back into the pot of simmering broth and stir well.
4. Add the diced tofu, chopped greens, green onions, soy sauce or tamari, rice vinegar, sesame oil, grated ginger, and minced garlic to the pot.
5. Let the soup simmer for about 5 minutes, until the tofu is heated through and the greens are wilted.
6. Taste the soup and adjust the seasoning with soy sauce or tamari, rice vinegar, and red pepper flakes if desired.
7. Serve the miso soup hot, garnished with fresh cilantro or parsley if desired.

Nutritional Information (per serving):

- Calories: 150
- Protein: 12g
- Total Fats: 7g
- Fiber: 5g
- Carbohydrates: 10g

Sweet Potato and Carrot Soup

Time to Prepare: 10 minutes
Cooking Time: 25 minutes
Number of Servings: 4 servings

Ingredients:

- 2 large sweet potatoes, peeled and diced
- 3 large carrots, peeled and chopped
- 1 onion, diced
- 3 cloves garlic, minced
- 4 cups of vegetable broth
- 1 teaspoon of ground turmeric
- 1/2 teaspoon of ground ginger
- Salt and pepper, to taste
- 2 tablespoons olive oil
- Fresh cilantro or parsley, for garnish (optional)

Instructions List:

1. In a large pot, heat the olive oil over medium heat. Add the diced onion and minced garlic. Sauté for 2-3 minutes until softened.
2. Add the diced sweet potatoes and chopped carrots to the pot. Stir to combine with the onion and garlic.
3. Pour in the vegetable broth, then add the ground turmeric and ground ginger. Season with salt and pepper to taste.
4. Bring the mixture to a boil, then reduce the heat to low. Cover and simmer for 20-25 minutes, or until the sweet potatoes and carrots are tender.
5. Once the vegetables are cooked, remove the pot from the heat. Use an immersion blender to puree the soup until smooth. Alternatively, carefully transfer the soup to a blender and blend until smooth, then return to the pot.
6. Taste and adjust seasoning if needed. If the soup is too thick, you can add more vegetable broth or water to reach your desired consistency.
7. Serve the soup hot, garnished with fresh cilantro or parsley if desired.

Nutritional Information (per serving):

- Calories: 187
- Protein: 3g
- Total Fats: 7g
- Fiber: 5g
- Carbohydrates: 29g

Broccoli and Kale Soup

Time to Prepare: 10 minutes
Cooking Time: 20 minutes
Number of Servings: 4 servings

Ingredients:

- 1 tablespoon olive oil
- 1 onion, chopped
- 2 cloves garlic, minced
- 1 head broccoli, chopped
- 2 cups of chopped kale
- 4 cups of vegetable broth
- 1 teaspoon of dried thyme
- Salt and pepper, to taste
- Juice of 1 lemon
- Fresh parsley, for garnish (optional)

Instructions List:

1. In a large pot, heat the olive oil over medium heat. Add the chopped onion and minced garlic. Sauté for 2-3 minutes until softened.
2. Add the chopped broccoli and kale to the pot. Stir to combine with the onion and garlic.
3. Pour in the vegetable broth and add the dried thyme. Season with salt and pepper to taste.
4. Bring the mixture to a boil, then reduce the heat to low. Cover and simmer for 15-20 minutes, or until the broccoli is tender.
5. Once the vegetables are cooked, remove the pot from the heat. Use an immersion blender to puree the soup until smooth. Alternatively, carefully transfer the soup to a blender and blend until smooth, then return to the pot.
6. Stir in the lemon juice.
7. Serve the soup hot, garnished with fresh parsley if desired.

Nutritional Information (per serving):

- Calories: 112
- Protein: 4g
- Total Fats: 4g
- Fiber: 5g
- Carbohydrates: 17g

Turmeric Ginger Vegetable Soup

Time to Prepare: 10 minutes
Cooking Time: 30 minutes
Number of Servings: 6

Ingredients:

- 1 tablespoon olive oil
- 1 onion, diced
- 3 cloves garlic, minced
- 1 tablespoon grated ginger
- 2 carrots, diced
- 2 celery stalks, diced
- 1 bell pepper, diced
- 1 zucchini, diced
- 1 cup of diced tomatoes
- 6 cups vegetable broth
- 1 teaspoon of ground turmeric
- 1/2 teaspoon of ground cumin
- 1/2 teaspoon of ground coriander
- Salt and pepper to taste
- Fresh cilantro or parsley for garnish (optional)

Instructions List:

1. Heat the olive oil in a large pot over medium heat.
2. Add the diced onion and cook until softened, about 5 minutes.
3. Stir in the minced garlic and grated ginger, and cook for another minute until fragrant.
4. Add the diced carrots, celery, bell pepper, and zucchini to the pot. Cook for 5-7 minutes, stirring occasionally, until the vegetables start to soften.
5. Stir in the diced tomatoes, vegetable broth, ground turmeric, ground cumin, and ground coriander.
6. Bring the soup to a simmer and let it cook for about 15-20 minutes, or until the vegetables are tender.
7. Season the soup with salt and pepper to taste.
8. Serve the turmeric ginger vegetable soup hot, garnished with fresh cilantro or parsley if desired.

Nutritional Information (per serving):

- Calories: 100
- Protein: 3g
- Total Fats: 3g

- Fiber: 4g
- Carbohydrates: 15g

Coconut Curry Butternut Squash Soup

Time to Prepare: 15 minutes
Cooking Time: 30 minutes
Number of Servings: 6 servings

Ingredients:

- 1 tablespoon coconut oil
- 1 onion, chopped
- 3 cloves garlic, minced
- 1 tablespoon curry powder
- 1 teaspoon of ground turmeric
- 1 teaspoon of ground cumin
- 1/2 teaspoon of ground cinnamon
- 1 butternut squash, peeled, seeded, and cubed
- 4 cups of vegetable broth
- 1 can (14 oz) coconut milk
- Salt and pepper, to taste
- Fresh cilantro, for garnish (optional)

Instructions List:

1. In a large pot, heat the coconut oil over medium heat. Add the chopped onion and minced garlic. Sauté for 2-3 minutes until softened.
2. Add the curry powder, turmeric, cumin, and cinnamon to the pot. Stir to combine with the onion and garlic, and cook for an additional 1-2 minutes until fragrant.
3. Add the cubed butternut squash to the pot, along with the vegetable broth. Bring to a boil, then reduce the heat to low. Cover and simmer for 20-25 minutes, or until the squash is tender.
4. Once the squash is cooked, remove the pot from the heat. Use an immersion blender to puree the soup until smooth. Alternatively, carefully transfer the soup to a blender and blend until smooth, then return to the pot.
5. Stir in the coconut milk and season with salt and pepper to taste.
6. Return the pot to the heat and simmer for an additional 5 minutes to heat through.
7. Serve the soup hot, garnished with fresh cilantro if desired.

Nutritional Information (per serving):

- Calories: 228
- Protein: 4g

- Total Fats: 18g
- Fiber: 6g
- Carbohydrates: 19g

Spiced Chickpea and Spinach Stew

Time to Prepare: 10 minutes
Cooking Time: 25 minutes
Number of Servings: 4 servings

Ingredients:

- 1 tablespoon olive oil
- 1 onion, chopped
- 3 cloves garlic, minced
- 1 teaspoon of ground cumin
- 1 teaspoon of ground coriander
- 1/2 teaspoon of smoked paprika
- 1/4 teaspoon of cayenne pepper (optional)
- 1 can (15 oz) chickpeas, drained and rinsed
- 1 can (14 oz) diced tomatoes
- 2 cups of vegetable broth
- 4 cups of fresh spinach leaves
- Salt and pepper, to taste
- Fresh cilantro, for garnish (optional)

Instructions List:

1. Heat the olive oil in a large pot over medium heat. Add the chopped onion and minced garlic. Sauté for 2-3 minutes until softened.
2. Add the ground cumin, ground coriander, smoked paprika, and cayenne pepper (if using) to the pot. Stir to combine with the onion and garlic, and cook for an additional 1-2 minutes until fragrant.
3. Add the chickpeas, diced tomatoes, and vegetable broth to the pot. Bring to a simmer and cook for 15 minutes, stirring occasionally.
4. Once the stew has simmered for 15 minutes, add the fresh spinach leaves to the pot. Stir until the spinach wilts and is incorporated into the stew.
5. Season the stew with salt and pepper to taste.
6. Serve the stew hot, garnished with fresh cilantro if desired.

Nutritional Information (per serving):

- Calories: 233
- Protein: 9g

- Total Fats: 7g
- Fiber: 10g
- Carbohydrates: 36g

Cauliflower Leek Soup

Time to Prepare: 10 minutes
Cooking Time: 25 minutes
Number of Servings: 4 servings

Ingredients:

- 1 tablespoon olive oil
- 2 leeks, white and light green parts only, chopped
- 3 cloves garlic, minced
- 1 medium head cauliflower, chopped into florets
- 4 cups of vegetable broth
- 1 teaspoon of dried thyme
- Salt and pepper, to taste
- Fresh parsley, for garnish (optional)

Instructions List:

1. Heat the olive oil in a large pot over medium heat. Add the chopped leeks and minced garlic. Sauté for 3-4 minutes until softened.
2. Add the cauliflower florets to the pot and cook for another 5 minutes, stirring occasionally.
3. Pour in the vegetable broth and add the dried thyme. Bring the soup to a simmer and cook for 15 minutes, or until the cauliflower is tender.
4. Using an immersion blender, blend the soup until smooth. Alternatively, transfer the soup in batches to a blender and blend until smooth, then return to the pot.
5. Season the soup with salt and pepper to taste.
6. Serve the soup hot, garnished with fresh parsley if desired.

Nutritional Information (per serving):

- Calories: 102
- Protein: 3g
- Total Fats: 4g
- Fiber: 4g
- Carbohydrates: 16g

Tomato and Red Pepper Soup

Time to Prepare: 10 minutes
Cooking Time: 30 minutes
Number of Servings: 4 servings

Ingredients:

- 1 tablespoon olive oil
- 1 onion, chopped
- 2 cloves garlic, minced
- 2 red bell peppers, seeded and chopped
- 4 large tomatoes, chopped
- 4 cups of vegetable broth
- 1 teaspoon of dried basil
- Salt and pepper, to taste
- Fresh basil leaves, for garnish (optional)

Instructions List:

1. Heat the olive oil in a large pot over medium heat. Add the chopped onion and minced garlic. Sauté for 3-4 minutes until softened.
2. Add the chopped red bell peppers and cook for another 5 minutes, stirring occasionally.
3. Stir in the chopped tomatoes and cook for 5 minutes.
4. Pour in the vegetable broth and add the dried basil. Bring the soup to a simmer and cook for 15 minutes.
5. Using an immersion blender, blend the soup until smooth. Alternatively, transfer the soup in batches to a blender and blend until smooth, then return to the pot.
6. Season the soup with salt and pepper to taste.
7. Serve the soup hot, garnished with fresh basil leaves if desired.

Nutritional Information (per serving):

- Calories: 94
- Protein: 2g
- Total Fats: 4g
- Fiber: 3g
- Carbohydrates: 14g

Zucchini and Basil Soup

Time to Prepare: 10 minutes
Cooking Time: 20 minutes
Number of Servings: 4

Ingredients:

- 1 tablespoon olive oil
- 1 onion, chopped
- 2 cloves garlic, minced
- 4 medium zucchinis, chopped
- 4 cups of vegetable broth
- 1/2 cup of fresh basil leaves
- Salt and pepper to taste
- Lemon wedges for serving (optional)

Instructions List:

1. In a large pot, heat the olive oil over medium heat.
2. Add the chopped onion and cook until softened, about 5 minutes.
3. Add the minced garlic and cook for another minute until fragrant.
4. Add the chopped zucchinis to the pot and cook for 5-7 minutes, stirring occasionally, until slightly softened.
5. Pour in the vegetable broth and bring the mixture to a simmer.
6. Let the soup simmer for about 10 minutes, or until the zucchinis are completely tender.
7. Stir in the fresh basil leaves and cook for another 2 minutes.
8. Remove the pot from heat and let the soup cool slightly.
9. Use an immersion blender to blend the soup until smooth.
10. Season the soup with salt and pepper to taste.
11. Serve the zucchini and basil soup hot, with lemon wedges for squeezing over the top if desired.

Nutritional Information (per serving):

- Calories: 80
- Protein: 2g
- Total Fats: 4g
- Fiber: 3g
- Carbohydrates: 10g

Mushroom and Barley Soup

Time to Prepare: 15 minutes
Cooking Time: 45 minutes
Number of Servings: 6

Ingredients:

- 2 tablespoons olive oil
- 1 onion, diced

- 3 cloves garlic, minced
- 3 carrots, diced
- 2 celery stalks, diced
- 500g mushrooms, sliced
- 1 cup of pearl barley, rinsed
- 6 cups vegetable broth
- 1 teaspoon of dried thyme
- 1 teaspoon of dried rosemary
- Salt and pepper to taste
- Fresh parsley for garnish (optional)

Instructions List:

1. Heat the olive oil in a large pot over medium heat.
2. Add the diced onion and cook until softened, about 5 minutes.
3. Add the minced garlic, diced carrots, and diced celery to the pot. Cook for another 5 minutes, stirring occasionally.
4. Add the sliced mushrooms and cook until they release their moisture and begin to brown, about 10 minutes.
5. Stir in the pearl barley, vegetable broth, dried thyme, and dried rosemary.
6. Bring the soup to a boil, then reduce the heat to low and let it simmer for about 30 minutes, or until the barley is tender.
7. Season the soup with salt and pepper to taste.
8. Serve the mushroom and barley soup hot, garnished with fresh parsley if desired.

Nutritional Information (per serving):

- Calories: 200
- Protein: 6g
- Total Fats: 6g
- Fiber: 6g
- Carbohydrates: 32g

Gingered Carrot Soup

Time to Prepare: 10 minutes
Cooking Time: 30 minutes
Number of Servings: 4

Ingredients:

- 1 tablespoon olive oil

- 1 onion, chopped
- 2 cloves garlic, minced
- 1 tablespoon fresh ginger, grated
- 1 kg carrots, peeled and chopped
- 4 cups of vegetable broth
- 1 cup of coconut milk
- Salt and pepper to taste
- Fresh cilantro for garnish (optional)

Instructions List:

1. Heat the olive oil in a large pot over medium heat.
2. Add the chopped onion and cook until softened, about 5 minutes.
3. Add the minced garlic and grated ginger, and cook for another minute until fragrant.
4. Add the chopped carrots and cook for 5 minutes, stirring occasionally.
5. Pour in the vegetable broth and bring the mixture to a boil.
6. Reduce the heat to low and let the soup simmer for about 20 minutes, or until the carrots are tender.
7. Stir in the coconut milk and let the soup heat through.
8. Remove the pot from heat and let the soup cool slightly.
9. Use an immersion blender to blend the soup until smooth.
10. Season the soup with salt and pepper to taste.
11. Serve the gingered carrot soup hot, garnished with fresh cilantro if desired.

Nutritional Information (per serving):

- Calories: 180
- Protein: 3g
- Total Fats: 10g
- Fiber: 5g
- Carbohydrates: 20g

Sweet Corn and Quinoa Soup

Time to Prepare: 10 minutes
Cooking Time: 25 minutes
Number of Servings: 4

Ingredients:

- 1 tablespoon olive oil
- 1 onion, chopped

- 2 cloves garlic, minced
- 2 cups of sweet corn kernels (fresh or frozen)
- 1/2 cup of quinoa, rinsed
- 4 cups of vegetable broth
- 1 cup of coconut milk
- 1 teaspoon of ground turmeric
- 1/2 teaspoon of ground cumin
- Salt and pepper to taste
- Fresh cilantro for garnish (optional)

Instructions List:
1. Heat the olive oil in a large pot over medium heat.
2. Add the chopped onion and cook until softened, about 5 minutes.
3. Add the minced garlic and cook for another minute until fragrant.
4. Stir in the sweet corn kernels and quinoa, and cook for 2-3 minutes.
5. Pour in the vegetable broth and bring the mixture to a boil.
6. Reduce the heat to low and let the soup simmer for about 20 minutes, or until the quinoa is tender.
7. Stir in the coconut milk, ground turmeric, and ground cumin, and let the soup heat through.
8. Season the soup with salt and pepper to taste.
9. Serve the sweet corn and quinoa soup hot, garnished with fresh cilantro if desired.

Nutritional Information (per serving):
- Calories: 220
- Protein: 6g
- Total Fats: 10g
- Fiber: 5g
- Carbohydrates: 28g

Red Lentil and Spinach Soup

Time to Prepare: 10 minutes
Cooking Time: 30 minutes
Number of Servings: 4

Ingredients:
- 1 tablespoon olive oil
- 1 onion, chopped
- 2 cloves garlic, minced

- 1 tablespoon fresh ginger, grated
- 1 cup of red lentils, rinsed
- 4 cups of vegetable broth
- 1 can (400g) diced tomatoes
- 2 cups of fresh spinach, chopped
- 1 teaspoon of ground cumin
- 1 teaspoon of ground coriander
- 1/2 teaspoon of ground turmeric
- 1/2 teaspoon of ground paprika
- Salt and pepper to taste
- Fresh lemon wedges for serving (optional)

Instructions List:
1. Heat the olive oil in a large pot over medium heat.
2. Add the chopped onion and cook until softened, about 5 minutes.
3. Add the minced garlic and grated ginger, and cook for another minute until fragrant.
4. Stir in the red lentils, vegetable broth, and diced tomatoes.
5. Add the ground cumin, ground coriander, ground turmeric, and ground paprika.
6. Bring the mixture to a boil, then reduce the heat to low and let it simmer for about 20 minutes, or until the lentils are tender.
7. Stir in the chopped spinach and cook for another 5 minutes, until the spinach is wilted.
8. Season the soup with salt and pepper to taste.
9. Serve the red lentil and spinach soup hot, with fresh lemon wedges for squeezing over the top if desired.

Nutritional Information (per serving):
- Calories: 210
- Protein: 12g
- Total Fats: 5g
- Fiber: 8g
- Carbohydrates: 30g

Chapter 4: Salads

Kale and Avocado Salad

Time to Prepare: 15 minutes
Cooking Time: 0 minutes
Number of Servings: 4

Ingredients:

- 1 bunch kale, stems removed and leaves chopped
- 1 avocado, diced
- 1/4 cup of red onion, thinly sliced
- 1/4 cup of cherry tomatoes, halved
- 1/4 cup of pumpkin seeds
- 1 lemon, juiced
- 2 tablespoons olive oil
- Salt and pepper to taste

Instructions List:

1. In a large bowl, add the chopped kale.
2. Drizzle the lemon juice and olive oil over the kale. Massage the kale with your hands for 2-3 minutes until it becomes tender.
3. Add the diced avocado, red onion, cherry tomatoes, and pumpkin seeds to the bowl.
4. Toss the salad gently to combine all ingredients.
5. Season with salt and pepper to taste.
6. Serve the kale and avocado salad immediately.

Nutritional Information (per serving):

- Calories: 180
- Protein: 4g
- Total Fats: 15g
- Fiber: 6g
- Carbohydrates: 11g

Rainbow Quinoa Salad

Time to Prepare: 15 minutes
Cooking Time: 15 minutes
Number of Servings: 4

Ingredients:

- 1 cup of quinoa, rinsed
- 2 cups of water
- 1 red bell pepper, diced
- 1 yellow bell pepper, diced
- 1 cup of cherry tomatoes, halved
- 1/2 cup of shredded purple cabbage
- 1/2 cup of grated carrots
- 1/4 cup of chopped fresh parsley
- 1/4 cup of chopped fresh cilantro
- 1/4 cup of olive oil
- 2 tablespoons lemon juice
- 1 tablespoon apple cider vinegar
- Salt and pepper to taste

Instructions List:

1. In a medium pot, bring the quinoa and water to a boil. Reduce the heat, cover, and simmer for about 15 minutes, or until the water is absorbed and the quinoa is tender. Let it cool.
2. In a large bowl, combine the cooked quinoa, red bell pepper, yellow bell pepper, cherry tomatoes, purple cabbage, carrots, parsley, and cilantro.
3. In a small bowl, whisk together the olive oil, lemon juice, apple cider vinegar, salt, and pepper.
4. Pour the dressing over the quinoa and vegetables, and toss to combine.
5. Serve the rainbow quinoa salad chilled or at room temperature.

Nutritional Information (per serving):

- Calories: 220
- Protein: 5g
- Total Fats: 12g
- Fiber: 5g
- Carbohydrates: 24g

Spinach and Strawberry Salad

Time to Prepare: 10 minutes
Cooking Time: 0 minutes
Number of Servings: 4

Ingredients:

- 6 cups fresh spinach, washed and dried
- 2 cups of strawberries, hulled and sliced

- 1/4 cup of red onion, thinly sliced
- 1/4 cup of sliced almonds
- 2 tablespoons balsamic vinegar
- 1 tablespoon olive oil
- 1 tablespoon maple syrup
- Salt and pepper to taste

Instructions List:

1. In a large bowl, combine the fresh spinach, sliced strawberries, red onion, and sliced almonds.
2. In a small bowl, whisk together the balsamic vinegar, olive oil, maple syrup, salt, and pepper.
3. Pour the dressing over the salad and toss gently to combine.
4. Serve the spinach and strawberry salad immediately.

Nutritional Information (per serving):

- Calories: 130
- Protein: 3g
- Total Fats: 7g
- Fiber: 4g
- Carbohydrates: 14g

Roasted Beet and Orange Salad

Time to Prepare: 15 minutes
Cooking Time: 45 minutes
Number of Servings: 4

Ingredients:

- 4 medium beets, peeled and diced
- 2 oranges, peeled and segmented
- 4 cups of mixed salad greens
- 1/4 cup of walnuts, chopped
- 2 tablespoons balsamic vinegar
- 2 tablespoons olive oil
- 1 teaspoon of maple syrup
- Salt and pepper to taste

Instructions List:

1. Preheat the oven to 400°F (200°C).

2. Place the diced beets on a baking sheet lined with parchment paper. Drizzle with olive oil and season with salt and pepper. Toss to coat evenly.
3. Roast the beets in the preheated oven for about 40-45 minutes, or until tender. Let them cool slightly.
4. In a large bowl, combine the roasted beets, orange segments, mixed salad greens, and chopped walnuts.
5. In a small bowl, whisk together the balsamic vinegar, olive oil, maple syrup, salt, and pepper to make the dressing.
6. Pour the dressing over the salad and toss gently to coat all ingredients.
7. Serve the roasted beet and orange salad immediately.

Nutritional Information (per serving):

- Calories: 200
- Protein: 4g
- Total Fats: 10g
- Fiber: 6g
- Carbohydrates: 25g

Cucumber and Tomato Salad with Mint

Time to Prepare: 10 minutes
Cooking Time: 0 minutes
Number of Servings: 4

Ingredients:

- 2 large cucumbers, diced
- 2 cups of cherry tomatoes, halved
- 1/4 cup of red onion, thinly sliced
- 2 tablespoons fresh mint leaves, chopped
- 2 tablespoons lemon juice
- 1 tablespoon olive oil
- Salt and pepper to taste

Instructions List:

1. In a large bowl, combine the diced cucumbers, cherry tomatoes, sliced red onion, and chopped mint leaves.
2. In a small bowl, whisk together the lemon juice, olive oil, salt, and pepper.
3. Pour the dressing over the salad and toss gently to coat all ingredients.
4. Serve the cucumber and tomato salad with mint immediately.

Nutritional Information (per serving):

- Calories: 60

- Protein: 2g
- Total Fats: 4g
- Fiber: 2g
- Carbohydrates: 8g

Arugula and Pear Salad

Time to Prepare: 10 minutes
Cooking Time: 0 minutes
Number of Servings: 4

Ingredients:

- 6 cups arugula
- 2 ripe pears, thinly sliced
- 1/4 cup of walnuts, chopped
- 1/4 cup of dried cranberries
- 2 tablespoons balsamic vinegar
- 1 tablespoon olive oil
- 1 teaspoon of maple syrup
- Salt and pepper to taste

Instructions List:

1. In a large bowl, combine the arugula, sliced pears, chopped walnuts, and dried cranberries.
2. In a small bowl, whisk together the balsamic vinegar, olive oil, maple syrup, salt, and pepper to make the dressing.
3. Pour the dressing over the salad and toss gently to coat all ingredients.
4. Serve the arugula and pear salad immediately.

Nutritional Information (per serving):

- Calories: 150
- Protein: 2g
- Total Fats: 8g
- Fiber: 4g
- Carbohydrates: 20g

Warm Lentil and Sweet Potato Salad

Time to Prepare: 15 minutes
Cooking Time: 30 minutes
Number of Servings: 4

Ingredients:

- 1 cup of green lentils, rinsed
- 2 medium sweet potatoes, peeled and diced
- 1 red bell pepper, diced
- 1/4 cup of red onion, finely chopped
- 2 tablespoons fresh parsley, chopped
- 2 tablespoons olive oil
- 1 tablespoon balsamic vinegar
- 1 teaspoon of Dijon mustard
- Salt and pepper to taste

Instructions List:

1. In a medium pot, bring the green lentils and 2 cups of water to a boil. Reduce the heat, cover, and simmer for about 20-25 minutes, or until the lentils are tender. Drain any excess water.
2. While the lentils are cooking, preheat the oven to 400°F (200°C).
3. Place the diced sweet potatoes on a baking sheet lined with parchment paper. Drizzle with olive oil, season with salt and pepper, and toss to coat evenly. Roast in the preheated oven for about 20-25 minutes, or until tender and slightly browned.
4. In a large bowl, combine the cooked lentils, roasted sweet potatoes, diced red bell pepper, chopped red onion, and chopped parsley.
5. In a small bowl, whisk together the olive oil, balsamic vinegar, Dijon mustard, salt, and pepper to make the dressing.
6. Pour the dressing over the salad and toss gently to coat all ingredients.
7. Serve the warm lentil and sweet potato salad immediately.

Nutritional Information (per serving):

- Calories: 280
- Protein: 10g
- Total Fats: 8g
- Fiber: 10g
- Carbohydrates: 40g

Broccoli and Cranberry Salad

Time to Prepare: 15 minutes
Cooking Time: 0 minutes
Number of Servings: 4

Ingredients:

- 4 cups of broccoli florets, blanched

- 1/2 cup of dried cranberries
- 1/4 cup of red onion, thinly sliced
- 1/4 cup of sunflower seeds
- 2 tablespoons apple cider vinegar
- 2 tablespoons olive oil
- 1 tablespoon maple syrup
- Salt and pepper to taste

Instructions List:

1. In a large bowl, combine the blanched broccoli florets, dried cranberries, sliced red onion, and sunflower seeds.
2. In a small bowl, whisk together the apple cider vinegar, olive oil, maple syrup, salt, and pepper to make the dressing.
3. Pour the dressing over the salad and toss gently to coat all ingredients.
4. Serve the broccoli and cranberry salad immediately.

Nutritional Information (per serving):

- Calories: 180
- Protein: 4g
- Total Fats: 9g
- Fiber: 5g
- Carbohydrates: 25g

Turmeric Cauliflower Rice Salad

Time to Prepare: 10 minutes
Cooking Time: 10 minutes
Number of Servings: 4

Ingredients:

- 1 medium head cauliflower, grated (or 4 cups of cauliflower rice)
- 1 tablespoon olive oil
- 1 teaspoon of ground turmeric
- 1/2 teaspoon of ground cumin
- 1/4 teaspoon of ground coriander
- 1/4 teaspoon of garlic powder
- Salt and pepper to taste
- 1/4 cup of fresh cilantro, chopped
- 1/4 cup of roasted cashews, chopped

- 1/4 cup of raisins

Instructions List:

1. Heat the olive oil in a large skillet over medium heat.
2. Add the grated cauliflower to the skillet and cook for 5-6 minutes, stirring occasionally, until the cauliflower is tender.
3. Stir in the ground turmeric, ground cumin, ground coriander, garlic powder, salt, and pepper. Cook for another 2-3 minutes, stirring constantly, to toast the spices.
4. Remove the skillet from heat and let the cauliflower rice cool slightly.
5. In a large bowl, combine the cooked cauliflower rice, chopped cilantro, chopped roasted cashews, and raisins. Toss gently to mix all ingredients.
6. Serve the turmeric cauliflower rice salad warm or at room temperature.

Nutritional Information (per serving):

- Calories: 120
- Protein: 4g
- Total Fats: 7g
- Fiber: 5g
- Carbohydrates: 14g

Asian Sesame Cabbage Salad

Time to Prepare: 15 minutes
Cooking Time: 0 minutes
Number of Servings: 4 servings

Ingredients:

- 1 small head green cabbage, thinly sliced
- 1 large carrot, julienned or grated
- 1/4 cup of chopped cilantro
- 2 green onions, thinly sliced
- 1/4 cup of toasted sesame seeds
- 1/4 cup of rice vinegar
- 2 tablespoons soy sauce or tamari
- 1 tablespoon maple syrup or agave syrup
- 1 tablespoon toasted sesame oil
- 1 teaspoon of grated ginger
- 1 clove garlic, minced
- Salt and pepper, to taste

- Optional: red pepper flakes, for added heat

Instructions List:

1. In a large mixing bowl, combine the sliced cabbage, julienned carrot, chopped cilantro, sliced green onions, and toasted sesame seeds.
2. In a small bowl, whisk together the rice vinegar, soy sauce or tamari, maple syrup or agave syrup, toasted sesame oil, grated ginger, minced garlic, salt, pepper, and red pepper flakes (if using).
3. Pour the dressing over the cabbage mixture and toss until everything is well coated.
4. Let the salad sit for about 10 minutes to allow the flavors to meld together.
5. Taste and adjust seasoning if needed.
6. Serve the Asian sesame cabbage salad as a side dish or as a light meal on its own.

Nutritional Information (per serving):

- Calories: 120
- Protein: 4g
- Total Fats: 6g
- Fiber: 5g
- Carbohydrates: 14g

Grilled Vegetable Salad

Time to Prepare: 15 minutes
Cooking Time: 15 minutes
Number of Servings: 4 servings

Ingredients:

- 2 medium zucchinis, sliced lengthwise
- 2 red bell peppers, seeded and quartered
- 1 large eggplant, sliced into rounds
- 1 red onion, sliced into rounds
- 2 tablespoons olive oil
- Salt and pepper, to taste
- 2 cups of mixed salad greens
- 1/4 cup of fresh basil leaves, torn
- 1/4 cup of toasted pine nuts or almonds

For the Dressing:

- 3 tablespoons balsamic vinegar
- 2 tablespoons olive oil
- 1 teaspoon of Dijon mustard

- 1 garlic clove, minced
- Salt and pepper, to taste

Instructions List:

1. Preheat a grill or grill pan over medium-high heat.
2. In a large bowl, toss the sliced zucchinis, red bell peppers, eggplant, and red onion with olive oil, salt, and pepper until evenly coated.
3. Grill the vegetables in batches, turning occasionally, until they are tender and have grill marks, about 3-4 minutes per side for the zucchinis and peppers, and 2-3 minutes per side for the eggplant and onions.
4. Remove the grilled vegetables from the grill and let them cool slightly.
5. Meanwhile, prepare the dressing by whisking together the balsamic vinegar, olive oil, Dijon mustard, minced garlic, salt, and pepper in a small bowl.
6. Arrange the mixed salad greens on a serving platter or individual plates.
7. Top the greens with the grilled vegetables, overlapping them slightly.
8. Drizzle the dressing over the salad and sprinkle with torn basil leaves and toasted pine nuts or almonds.
9. Serve the grilled vegetable salad immediately.

Nutritional Information (per serving):

- Calories: 220
- Protein: 5g
- Total Fats: 16g
- Fiber: 7g
- Carbohydrates: 18g

Mediterranean Farro Salad

Time to Prepare: 15 minutes
Cooking Time: 25 minutes
Number of Servings: 6 servings

Ingredients:

- 1 cup of farro, rinsed
- 2 cups of vegetable broth
- 1 cup of cherry tomatoes, halved
- 1 cucumber, diced
- 1/2 red onion, finely chopped
- 1/2 cup of Kalamata olives, pitted and halved
- 1/4 cup of fresh parsley, chopped
- 1/4 cup of fresh mint, chopped

- 1/4 cup of extra virgin olive oil
- 2 tablespoons lemon juice
- 1 garlic clove, minced
- Salt and pepper, to taste

Instructions List:

1. In a medium saucepan, combine the farro and vegetable broth. Bring to a boil over medium-high heat.
2. Reduce the heat to low, cover, and simmer for 20-25 minutes, or until the farro is tender and the liquid is absorbed. Remove from heat and let it cool slightly.
3. In a large mixing bowl, combine the cooked farro, cherry tomatoes, cucumber, red onion, Kalamata olives, parsley, and mint.
4. In a small bowl, whisk together the extra virgin olive oil, lemon juice, minced garlic, salt, and pepper to make the dressing.
5. Pour the dressing over the farro salad and toss until everything is evenly coated.
6. Taste and adjust seasoning if necessary.
7. Serve the Mediterranean farro salad immediately or refrigerate for later.

Nutritional Information (per serving):

- Calories: 270
- Protein: 5g
- Total Fats: 12g
- Fiber: 6g
- Carbohydrates: 36g

Mango Black Bean Salad

Time to Prepare: 15 minutes
Cooking Time: 0 minutes
Number of Servings: 4 servings

Ingredients:

- 1 can (15 ounces) black beans, rinsed and drained
- 1 ripe mango, diced
- 1 red bell pepper, diced
- 1/2 red onion, finely chopped
- 1/4 cup of fresh cilantro, chopped
- Juice of 1 lime
- 2 tablespoons extra virgin olive oil
- 1 teaspoon of ground cumin

- Salt and pepper, to taste
- Optional: diced avocado for garnish

Instructions List:

1. In a large mixing bowl, combine the black beans, diced mango, red bell pepper, red onion, and chopped cilantro.
2. In a small bowl, whisk together the lime juice, extra virgin olive oil, ground cumin, salt, and pepper to make the dressing.
3. Pour the dressing over the salad ingredients and toss gently until everything is well mixed.
4. Taste and adjust seasoning if necessary.
5. Garnish with diced avocado, if desired.
6. Serve immediately or refrigerate until ready to serve.

Nutritional Information (per serving):

- Calories: 230
- Protein: 6g
- Total Fats: 8g
- Fiber: 8g
- Carbohydrates: 34g

Spicy Thai Peanut Noodle Salad

Time to Prepare: 20 minutes
Cooking Time: 10 minutes
Number of Servings: 4 servings

Ingredients:

- 8 ounces whole grain spaghetti or rice noodles
- 1 red bell pepper, thinly sliced
- 1 large carrot, julienned
- 1 cup of shredded red cabbage
- 1/4 cup of chopped green onions
- 1/4 cup of chopped fresh cilantro
- 1/4 cup of chopped peanuts
- 2 tablespoons sesame seeds (optional, for garnish)

For the Spicy Peanut Sauce:

- 1/4 cup of creamy peanut butter
- 2 tablespoons soy sauce (or tamari for gluten-free)
- 2 tablespoons lime juice

- 2 tablespoons maple syrup
- 1 tablespoon sesame oil
- 1 tablespoon rice vinegar
- 1 teaspoon of grated ginger
- 1 clove garlic, minced
- 1 teaspoon of Sriracha sauce (adjust to taste)
- Water, as needed to thin the sauce

Instructions List:

1. Cook the noodles according to package instructions until al dente. Drain and rinse with cold water to stop cooking. Set aside.
2. In a large mixing bowl, combine the cooked noodles, sliced red bell pepper, julienned carrot, shredded red cabbage, chopped green onions, and chopped cilantro.
3. In a separate bowl, whisk together all the ingredients for the spicy peanut sauce until smooth. Add water gradually to thin the sauce to your desired consistency.
4. Pour the spicy peanut sauce over the noodle and vegetable mixture. Toss until everything is evenly coated with the sauce.
5. Garnish with chopped peanuts and sesame seeds, if desired.
6. Serve immediately or refrigerate until ready to serve.

Nutritional Information (per serving):

- Calories: 380
- Protein: 12g
- Total Fats: 18g
- Fiber: 8g
- Carbohydrates: 47g

Chapter 5: Main Dishes

Chickpea and Spinach Patties

Time to Prepare: 15 minutes
Cooking Time: 15 minutes
Number of Servings: 4

Ingredients:

- 1 can (15 ounces) chickpeas, drained and rinsed
- 2 cups of fresh spinach, chopped
- 1/4 cup of red onion, finely chopped
- 2 cloves garlic, minced
- 2 tablespoons nutritional yeast
- 1 tablespoon ground flaxseeds
- 2 tablespoons water
- 1 teaspoon of ground cumin
- 1 teaspoon of ground coriander
- 1/2 teaspoon of smoked paprika
- Salt and pepper to taste
- 2 tablespoons olive oil (for cooking)

Instructions List:

1. In a food processor, combine the chickpeas, chopped spinach, red onion, minced garlic, nutritional yeast, ground flaxseeds, water, ground cumin, ground coriander, smoked paprika, salt, and pepper. Pulse until well mixed but still slightly chunky.
2. Shape the mixture into 8 patties, using your hands to firmly press them together.
3. Heat the olive oil in a large skillet over medium heat.
4. Add the patties to the skillet and cook for about 5-6 minutes on each side, or until golden brown and crispy.
5. Once cooked, transfer the patties to a plate lined with paper towels to absorb any excess oil.
6. Serve the chickpea and spinach patties warm, optionally with your favorite dipping sauce or on a salad.

Nutritional Information (per serving):

- Calories: 220
- Protein: 9g
- Total Fats: 9g
- Fiber: 8g
- Carbohydrates: 27g

Black Bean and Sweet Potato Burgers

Time to Prepare: 20 minutes
Cooking Time: 25 minutes
Number of Servings: 4

Ingredients:

- 1 can (15 ounces) black beans, drained and rinsed
- 1 medium sweet potato, peeled and grated
- 1/4 cup of red onion, finely chopped
- 2 cloves garlic, minced
- 1 tablespoon ground flaxseeds
- 2 tablespoons water
- 1 teaspoon of ground cumin
- 1 teaspoon of smoked paprika
- Salt and pepper to taste
- 1/4 cup of breadcrumbs (gluten-free if needed)
- 2 tablespoons olive oil (for cooking)

Instructions List:

1. In a large bowl, mash the black beans with a fork until mostly smooth.
2. Add the grated sweet potato, chopped red onion, minced garlic, ground flaxseeds, water, ground cumin, smoked paprika, salt, and pepper to the bowl. Mix until well mixed.
3. Stir in the breadcrumbs until the mixture holds together well. If it's too dry, you can add a little more water.
4. Divide the mixture into 4 equal portions and shape each portion into a patty.
5. Heat the olive oil in a large skillet over medium heat.
6. Add the patties to the skillet and cook for about 5-6 minutes on each side, or until golden brown and crispy.
7. Once cooked, transfer the burgers to a plate lined with paper towels to absorb any excess oil.
8. Serve the black bean and sweet potato burgers warm, optionally on burger buns with your favorite toppings.

Nutritional Information (per serving):

- Calories: 260
- Protein: 9g
- Total Fats: 7g
- Fiber: 9g
- Carbohydrates: 42g

BBQ Jackfruit Sandwiches

Time to Prepare: 15 minutes
Cooking Time: 25 minutes
Number of Servings: 4

Ingredients:

- 2 cans (20 ounces total) young green jackfruit in water or brine, drained and rinsed
- 1 cup of barbecue sauce (look for a plant-based, low-sugar option)
- 1/2 cup of vegetable broth
- 1 tablespoon olive oil
- 1/2 teaspoon of garlic powder
- 1/2 teaspoon of smoked paprika
- 1/4 teaspoon of chili powder
- Salt and pepper to taste
- 4 whole grain burger buns
- Optional toppings: sliced red onion, avocado, lettuce, tomato

Instructions List:

1. Use your hands or a fork to shred the jackfruit into smaller pieces.
2. In a large skillet, heat the olive oil over medium heat. Add the shredded jackfruit and cook for 5 minutes, stirring occasionally.
3. In a small bowl, mix together the barbecue sauce, vegetable broth, garlic powder, smoked paprika, chili powder, salt, and pepper.
4. Pour the barbecue sauce mixture over the jackfruit in the skillet. Stir well to combine.
5. Reduce the heat to low, cover, and simmer for 20 minutes, stirring occasionally, until the jackfruit is tender and the sauce has thickened.
6. Toast the burger buns if desired.
7. Spoon the BBQ jackfruit mixture onto the bottom halves of the burger buns. Add any desired toppings, then cover with the top halves of the buns.
8. Serve the BBQ jackfruit sandwiches hot.

Nutritional Information (per serving):

- Calories: 380
- Protein: 5g
- Total Fats: 6g
- Fiber: 8g
- Carbohydrates: 76g

Vegan Meatloaf with Lentils and Walnuts

Time to Prepare: 20 minutes
Cooking Time: 45 minutes
Number of Servings: 6

Ingredients:

- 1 cup of cooked green lentils
- 1 cup of walnuts, finely chopped
- 1 small onion, finely chopped
- 2 cloves garlic, minced
- 1 celery stalk, finely chopped
- 1 carrot, grated
- 1 cup of rolled oats
- 1/4 cup of tomato paste
- 2 tablespoons soy sauce or tamari
- 1 tablespoon Dijon mustard
- 1 tablespoon ground flaxseeds
- 3 tablespoons water
- 1 teaspoon of dried thyme
- 1 teaspoon of dried oregano
- 1/2 teaspoon of smoked paprika
- Salt and pepper to taste
- Optional glaze: 1/4 cup of ketchup mixed with 1 tablespoon maple syrup

Instructions List:

1. Preheat the oven to 350°F (175°C). Lightly grease a loaf pan with olive oil or line it with parchment paper.
2. In a small bowl, mix together the ground flaxseeds and water. Let it sit for 5 minutes to thicken and form a flax "egg".
3. In a large mixing bowl, combine the cooked lentils, chopped walnuts, finely chopped onion, minced garlic, finely chopped celery, grated carrot, rolled oats, tomato paste, soy sauce or tamari, Dijon mustard, thyme, oregano, smoked paprika, salt, pepper, and the flax "egg". Mix until well mixed.
4. Press the mixture into the prepared loaf pan, smoothing the top with a spoon or spatula.
5. If using the optional glaze, spread it evenly over the top of the meatloaf.
6. Bake in the preheated oven for 40-45 minutes, or until the top is golden brown and the meatloaf is firm to the touch.
7. Allow the meatloaf to cool for a few minutes before slicing and serving.

Nutritional Information (per serving):

- Calories: 320

- Protein: 13g
- Total Fats: 16g
- Fiber: 8g
- Carbohydrates: 35g

Seitan Stir-Fry with Vegetables

Time to Prepare: 15 minutes
Cooking Time: 15 minutes
Number of Servings: 4

Ingredients:

- 1 package (8 ounces) seitan, sliced or cubed
- 2 tablespoons soy sauce or tamari
- 1 tablespoon maple syrup
- 1 tablespoon sesame oil
- 1 tablespoon cornstarch
- 2 tablespoons water
- 1 tablespoon olive oil
- 2 cloves garlic, minced
- 1 inch piece of ginger, minced
- 1 red bell pepper, sliced
- 1 yellow bell pepper, sliced
- 1 small broccoli crown, cut into florets
- 1 medium carrot, sliced
- 1 cup of snap peas
- Salt and pepper to taste
- Cooked rice or noodles, for serving

Instructions List:

1. In a small bowl, mix together the soy sauce or tamari, maple syrup, sesame oil, cornstarch, and water to make the sauce. Set aside.
2. Heat the olive oil in a large skillet or wok over medium-high heat.
3. Add the minced garlic and ginger to the skillet and cook for 1 minute, or until fragrant.
4. Add the sliced or cubed seitan to the skillet and cook for 2-3 minutes, stirring occasionally, until lightly browned.
5. Add the sliced bell peppers, broccoli florets, sliced carrot, and snap peas to the skillet. Cook for 5-6 minutes, stirring frequently, until the vegetables are tender-crisp.

6. Pour the sauce over the seitan and vegetables in the skillet. Stir well to coat everything evenly.
7. Cook for another 2-3 minutes, or until the sauce has thickened slightly and everything is heated through.
8. Season with salt and pepper to taste.
9. Serve the seitan stir-fry with vegetables hot over cooked rice or noodles.

Nutritional Information (per serving):

- Calories: 280
- Protein: 20g
- Total Fats: 8g
- Fiber: 6g
- Carbohydrates: 30g

Tempeh Tacos with Avocado

Time to Prepare: 15 minutes
Cooking Time: 15 minutes
Number of Servings: 4

Ingredients:

- 1 package (8 ounces) tempeh, crumbled
- 2 tablespoons olive oil
- 1 small onion, diced
- 2 cloves garlic, minced
- 1 tablespoon chili powder
- 1 teaspoon of ground cumin
- 1/2 teaspoon of smoked paprika
- Salt and pepper to taste
- 1/4 cup of water or vegetable broth
- 8 small corn tortillas
- 1 ripe avocado, sliced
- Optional toppings: shredded lettuce, diced tomatoes, sliced jalapeños, salsa, lime wedges

Instructions List:

1. Heat 1 tablespoon of olive oil in a large skillet over medium heat.
2. Add the diced onion and minced garlic to the skillet. Cook for 2-3 minutes until softened.
3. Add the crumbled tempeh to the skillet along with the chili powder, ground cumin, smoked paprika, salt, and pepper. Stir to combine.
4. Pour in the water or vegetable broth and stir well. Cook for 5-7 minutes, stirring occasionally, until the tempeh is heated through and the liquid has evaporated.

5. While the tempeh is cooking, warm the corn tortillas in a separate skillet or in the oven.
6. Once the tempeh mixture is ready, assemble the tacos by spooning some of the mixture onto each warmed tortilla.
7. Top each taco with slices of avocado and any desired toppings.
8. Serve the tempeh tacos with avocado immediately, optionally with lime wedges on the side.

Nutritional Information (per serving):

- Calories: 320
- Protein: 15g
- Total Fats: 18g
- Fiber: 8g
- Carbohydrates: 30g

Portobello Mushroom Steaks

Time to Prepare: 10 minutes
Cooking Time: 15 minutes
Number of Servings: 2

Ingredients:

- 2 large portobello mushrooms, stems removed
- 2 tablespoons balsamic vinegar
- 2 tablespoons soy sauce or tamari
- 2 cloves garlic, minced
- 1 tablespoon olive oil
- 1 teaspoon of dried thyme
- Salt and pepper to taste
- Optional toppings: chopped fresh herbs (such as parsley or rosemary)

Instructions List:

1. In a small bowl, whisk together the balsamic vinegar, soy sauce or tamari, minced garlic, olive oil, dried thyme, salt, and pepper to make the marinade.
2. Place the portobello mushrooms in a shallow dish or a resealable plastic bag. Pour the marinade over the mushrooms, making sure they are well coated. Allow them to marinate for at least 30 minutes, or up to 2 hours in the refrigerator.
3. Preheat the grill or grill pan to medium-high heat.
4. Remove the mushrooms from the marinade and discard any excess marinade.
5. Place the mushrooms on the grill or grill pan, gill-side down. Cook for 5-7 minutes, then flip and cook for another 5-7 minutes, or until tender and slightly charred.
6. Remove the mushrooms from the grill and let them rest for a few minutes before serving.

7. Optionally, sprinkle the cooked mushrooms with chopped fresh herbs before serving.
8. Serve the portobello mushroom steaks hot.

Nutritional Information (per serving):

- Calories: 90
- Protein: 5g
- Total Fats: 5g
- Fiber: 3g
- Carbohydrates: 9g

Chickpea and Quinoa Stuffed Peppers

Time to Prepare: 15 minutes
Cooking Time: 40 minutes
Number of Servings: 4

Ingredients:

- 4 large bell peppers, any color
- 1 cup of cooked quinoa
- 1 can (15 ounces) chickpeas, drained and rinsed
- 1 cup of diced tomatoes
- 1/2 cup of diced onion
- 2 cloves garlic, minced
- 1 teaspoon of ground cumin
- 1 teaspoon of smoked paprika
- Salt and pepper to taste
- 1/4 cup of chopped fresh parsley or cilantro
- Optional toppings: avocado slices, vegan cheese, hot sauce

Instructions List:

1. Preheat the oven to 375°F (190°C). Lightly grease a baking dish.
2. Slice the tops off the bell peppers and remove the seeds and membranes. Place the peppers upright in the prepared baking dish.
3. In a large mixing bowl, combine the cooked quinoa, chickpeas, diced tomatoes, diced onion, minced garlic, ground cumin, smoked paprika, salt, pepper, and chopped fresh parsley or cilantro. Mix well to combine.
4. Spoon the quinoa and chickpea mixture into each bell pepper until they are full.
5. Cover the baking dish with foil and bake in the preheated oven for 25-30 minutes, or until the peppers are tender.
6. Remove the foil and bake for an additional 10 minutes, or until the tops are slightly golden.

7. Remove the stuffed peppers from the oven and let them cool for a few minutes before serving.
8. Optionally, top each stuffed pepper with avocado slices, vegan cheese, or hot sauce before serving.

Nutritional Information (per serving):

- Calories: 280
- Protein: 11g
- Total Fats: 4g
- Fiber: 9g
- Carbohydrates: 50g

Vegan Shepherd's Pie

Time to Prepare: 20 minutes
Cooking Time: 40 minutes
Number of Servings: 6

Ingredients:

- 4 large potatoes, peeled and diced
- 2 tablespoons olive oil
- 1 onion, chopped
- 2 cloves garlic, minced
- 2 carrots, diced
- 1 cup of frozen peas
- 1 cup of cooked lentils
- 1 cup of vegetable broth
- 2 tablespoons tomato paste
- 1 teaspoon of dried thyme
- 1 teaspoon of dried rosemary
- Salt and pepper to taste

Instructions List:

1. Preheat the oven to 375°F (190°C). Lightly grease a 9x13-inch baking dish.
2. Place the diced potatoes in a large pot of water. Bring to a boil and cook for 15-20 minutes, or until tender. Drain the potatoes and set aside.
3. In a large skillet, heat the olive oil over medium heat. Add the chopped onion and minced garlic, and cook for 2-3 minutes until softened.
4. Add the diced carrots to the skillet and cook for another 5 minutes, stirring occasionally.
5. Stir in the frozen peas, cooked lentils, vegetable broth, tomato paste, dried thyme, dried rosemary, salt, and pepper. Cook for an additional 5 minutes, allowing the flavors to meld together.

6. Transfer the lentil mixture to the prepared baking dish and spread it out evenly.
7. Mash the cooked potatoes with a potato masher or fork until smooth. Spread the mashed potatoes evenly over the lentil mixture in the baking dish.
8. Place the baking dish in the preheated oven and bake for 25-30 minutes, or until the mashed potatoes are lightly golden on top.
9. Remove from the oven and let it cool for a few minutes before serving.

Nutritional Information (per serving):

- Calories: 280
- Protein: 9g
- Total Fats: 5g
- Fiber: 8g
- Carbohydrates: 50g

Grilled Tofu with Chimichurri Sauce

Time to Prepare: 15 minutes
Cooking Time: 10 minutes
Number of Servings: 4

Ingredients:

- 1 block (14 ounces) firm tofu, pressed and drained
- 2 tablespoons olive oil
- Salt and pepper to taste
- Chimichurri Sauce:
    - 1 cup of fresh parsley, chopped
    - 1/4 cup of fresh cilantro, chopped
    - 2 cloves garlic, minced
    - 2 tablespoons red wine vinegar
    - 1/4 cup of olive oil
    - Salt and pepper to taste
    - Optional: red pepper flakes, for heat

Instructions List:

1. Preheat the grill or grill pan over medium-high heat.
2. Cut the pressed tofu into 1/2-inch thick slices and pat them dry with a paper towel.
3. Brush both sides of the tofu slices with olive oil and season with salt and pepper.
4. Place the tofu slices on the grill and cook for 4-5 minutes on each side, or until grill marks appear and the tofu is heated through.

5. While the tofu is grilling, prepare the chimichurri sauce. In a small bowl, combine the chopped parsley, chopped cilantro, minced garlic, red wine vinegar, olive oil, salt, pepper, and optional red pepper flakes. Mix well to combine.

6. Once the tofu is done grilling, transfer it to a serving plate and drizzle the chimichurri sauce over the top.

7. Serve the grilled tofu with chimichurri sauce immediately.

Nutritional Information (per serving):

- Calories: 230
- Protein: 11g
- Total Fats: 18g
- Fiber: 2g
- Carbohydrates: 7g

Eggplant Rollatini with Cashew Ricotta

Time to Prepare: 30 minutes
Cooking Time: 30 minutes
Number of Servings: 4

Ingredients:

- 2 large eggplants, thinly sliced lengthwise
- 2 tablespoons olive oil
- Salt and pepper to taste
- Cashew Ricotta:
    - 1 cup of raw cashews, soaked in water for 2-4 hours or overnight
    - 2 tablespoons nutritional yeast
    - 1 tablespoon lemon juice
    - 2 cloves garlic, minced
    - 1/4 teaspoon of salt
- Marinara Sauce:
    - 2 cups of tomato sauce
    - 1 teaspoon of dried basil
    - 1 teaspoon of dried oregano
    - 1/2 teaspoon of garlic powder
    - Salt and pepper to taste
- Optional: chopped fresh basil or parsley for garnish

Instructions List:

1. Preheat the oven to 375°F (190°C). Lightly grease a baking dish.

2. Place the thinly sliced eggplants on a baking sheet. Brush both sides of the eggplant slices with olive oil and season with salt and pepper.

3. Roast the eggplant slices in the preheated oven for 15-20 minutes, or until tender and slightly golden.

4. While the eggplant is roasting, prepare the cashew ricotta. Drain the soaked cashews and place them in a food processor or blender. Add the nutritional yeast, lemon juice, minced garlic, and salt. Blend until smooth and creamy. Set aside.

5. In a small saucepan, heat the tomato sauce over medium heat. Stir in the dried basil, dried oregano, garlic powder, salt, and pepper. Simmer for 5-10 minutes, stirring occasionally, until heated through.

6. Remove the roasted eggplant slices from the oven and let them cool slightly.

7. Spoon a dollop of cashew ricotta onto each eggplant slice and spread it evenly. Roll up the eggplant slices and place them seam-side down in the prepared baking dish.

8. Pour the marinara sauce over the rolled eggplant slices in the baking dish.

9. Bake in the preheated oven for 15-20 minutes, or until the sauce is bubbly.

10. Remove from the oven and let it cool for a few minutes before serving. Optionally, garnish with chopped fresh basil or parsley.

Nutritional Information (per serving):

- Calories: 320
- Protein: 10g
- Total Fats: 20g
- Fiber: 8g
- Carbohydrates: 30g

Spicy Lentil and Vegetable Stew

Time to Prepare: 15 minutes
Cooking Time: 40 minutes
Number of Servings: 6

Ingredients:

- 1 cup of dried green lentils, rinsed
- 1 tablespoon olive oil
- 1 onion, diced
- 2 cloves garlic, minced
- 2 carrots, diced
- 2 stalks celery, diced
- 1 bell pepper, diced
- 1 zucchini, diced
- 1 can (14 ounces) diced tomatoes

- 4 cups of vegetable broth
- 1 teaspoon of ground cumin
- 1 teaspoon of paprika
- 1/2 teaspoon of chili powder
- Salt and pepper to taste
- Fresh cilantro or parsley, for garnish (optional)

Instructions List:

1. In a large pot, heat the olive oil over medium heat. Add the diced onion and minced garlic, and sauté for 2-3 minutes until softened.
2. Add the diced carrots, celery, bell pepper, and zucchini to the pot. Cook for another 5 minutes, stirring occasionally.
3. Stir in the rinsed lentils, diced tomatoes, vegetable broth, ground cumin, paprika, chili powder, salt, and pepper.
4. Bring the stew to a boil, then reduce the heat to low. Cover and simmer for 30 minutes, or until the lentils and vegetables are tender.
5. Taste and adjust the seasoning if needed.
6. Serve the spicy lentil and vegetable stew hot, garnished with fresh cilantro or parsley if desired.

Nutritional Information (per serving):

- Calories: 220
- Protein: 12g
- Total Fats: 4g
- Fiber: 10g
- Carbohydrates: 34g

Pulled Jackfruit Tacos

Time to Prepare: 15 minutes
Cooking Time: 25 minutes
Number of Servings: 4

Ingredients:

- 2 cans (20 ounces each) young green jackfruit in water or brine, drained and rinsed
- 1 tablespoon olive oil
- 1 onion, diced
- 2 cloves garlic, minced
- 1 bell pepper, diced
- 1 teaspoon of ground cumin
- 1 teaspoon of smoked paprika

- 1/2 teaspoon of chili powder
- Salt and pepper to taste
- 1 cup of tomato sauce
- 2 tablespoons tomato paste
- 2 tablespoons apple cider vinegar
- 2 tablespoons maple syrup or agave nectar
- 8 small corn or flour tortillas
- Optional toppings: diced avocado, shredded lettuce, chopped cilantro, lime wedges

Instructions List:

1. Shred the jackfruit using your fingers or a fork to separate the fibers.
2. Heat the olive oil in a large skillet over medium heat. Add the diced onion and minced garlic, and cook until softened, about 3-4 minutes.
3. Add the shredded jackfruit and diced bell pepper to the skillet. Cook for 5-7 minutes, stirring occasionally, until the jackfruit starts to brown.
4. Stir in the ground cumin, smoked paprika, chili powder, salt, and pepper, and cook for another minute until fragrant.
5. Add the tomato sauce, tomato paste, apple cider vinegar, and maple syrup to the skillet. Stir well to combine.
6. Reduce the heat to low, cover, and simmer for 10-15 minutes, stirring occasionally, until the jackfruit mixture thickens and resembles pulled pork.
7. Warm the tortillas in a dry skillet or microwave.
8. To serve, spoon the pulled jackfruit mixture onto the warmed tortillas. Top with diced avocado, shredded lettuce, chopped cilantro, and a squeeze of lime juice if desired.
9. Serve the pulled jackfruit tacos immediately.

Nutritional Information (per serving):

- Calories: 320
- Protein: 5g
- Total Fats: 8g
- Fiber: 6g
- Carbohydrates: 60g

Vegan Tuna Salad with Chickpeas

Time to Prepare: 10 minutes
Cooking Time: 0 minutes
Number of Servings: 4

Ingredients:

- 2 cans (15 ounces each) chickpeas, drained and rinsed
- 1/4 cup of vegan mayonnaise
- 2 tablespoons Dijon mustard
- 2 tablespoons lemon juice
- 2 tablespoons finely chopped red onion
- 2 tablespoons chopped dill pickles
- 1 tablespoon nutritional yeast
- 1 teaspoon of kelp powder (for seafood flavor, optional)
- Salt and pepper to taste
- 4 leaves lettuce
- 4 whole grain bread slices

Instructions List:

1. In a large bowl, mash the chickpeas with a fork or potato masher until they reach your desired consistency.
2. Add the vegan mayonnaise, Dijon mustard, lemon juice, chopped red onion, chopped dill pickles, nutritional yeast, and kelp powder (if using) to the bowl with the mashed chickpeas. Mix well to combine.
3. Season the vegan tuna salad with salt and pepper to taste.
4. To assemble the sandwiches, place a leaf of lettuce on each slice of whole grain bread.
5. Divide the vegan tuna salad evenly among the sandwiches, spreading it over the lettuce leaves.
6. Top each sandwich with another slice of bread to form a sandwich.
7. Serve the vegan tuna salad sandwiches immediately, or wrap them tightly in foil or plastic wrap and refrigerate until ready to serve.

Nutritional Information (per serving):

- Calories: 290
- Protein: 12g
- Total Fats: 8g
- Fiber: 9g
- Carbohydrates: 42g

Watermelon Poke Bowl

Time to Prepare: 15 minutes
Cooking Time: 0 minutes
Number of Servings: 2

Ingredients:

- 2 cups of cooked sushi rice, cooled

- 2 cups of cubed seedless watermelon
- 1 avocado, diced
- 1/4 cup of sliced cucumber
- 1/4 cup of sliced radishes
- 2 tablespoons chopped green onions
- 2 tablespoons soy sauce or tamari
- 1 tablespoon sesame oil
- 1 tablespoon rice vinegar
- 1 teaspoon of grated ginger
- 1 teaspoon of sesame seeds
- 1/2 teaspoon of sriracha (optional)
- Nori strips, for garnish
- Pickled ginger, for serving (optional)
- Wasabi, for serving (optional)

Instructions List:

1. In a small bowl, whisk together the soy sauce or tamari, sesame oil, rice vinegar, grated ginger, sesame seeds, and sriracha (if using) to make the dressing.
2. In two serving bowls, divide the cooked sushi rice evenly.
3. Top the rice with cubed watermelon, diced avocado, sliced cucumber, sliced radishes, and chopped green onions.
4. Drizzle the dressing over the poke bowls.
5. Garnish with nori strips.
6. Serve the watermelon poke bowls immediately, with pickled ginger and wasabi on the side if desired.

Nutritional Information (per serving):

- Calories: 420
- Protein: 6g
- Total Fats: 16g
- Fiber: 8g
- Carbohydrates: 64g

Chapter 6: Snacks & Sides

Roasted Chickpeas

Time to Prepare: 5 minutes
Cooking Time: 40 minutes
Number of Servings: 4

Ingredients:

- 2 cans (15 ounces each) chickpeas, drained and rinsed
- 2 tablespoons olive oil
- 1 teaspoon of smoked paprika
- 1 teaspoon of ground cumin
- 1/2 teaspoon of garlic powder
- 1/2 teaspoon of onion powder
- 1/4 teaspoon of cayenne pepper (optional)
- Salt to taste

Instructions List:

1. Preheat your oven to 400°F (200°C). Line a baking sheet with parchment paper or lightly grease it.
2. Pat the chickpeas dry with a paper towel to remove excess moisture.
3. In a large bowl, toss the chickpeas with olive oil, smoked paprika, ground cumin, garlic powder, onion powder, and cayenne pepper (if using) until evenly coated.
4. Spread the seasoned chickpeas in a single layer on the prepared baking sheet.
5. Roast in the preheated oven for 30-40 minutes, stirring halfway through, until the chickpeas are golden brown and crispy.
6. Remove from the oven and let cool slightly before serving.
7. Season with salt to taste.
8. Serve the roasted chickpeas as a crunchy snack or as a topping for salads and bowls.

Nutritional Information (per serving):

- Calories: 220
- Protein: 8g
- Total Fats: 8g
- Fiber: 6g
- Carbohydrates: 28g

Baked Sweet Potato Fries

Time to Prepare: 10 minutes
Cooking Time: 25 minutes
Number of Servings: 4

Ingredients:

- 2 large sweet potatoes, scrubbed and cut into fries
- 2 tablespoons olive oil
- 1 teaspoon of garlic powder
- 1 teaspoon of paprika
- 1/2 teaspoon of onion powder
- 1/2 teaspoon of smoked paprika
- Salt and black pepper to taste

Instructions List:

1. Preheat your oven to 425°F (220°C). Line a baking sheet with parchment paper or lightly grease it.
2. In a large bowl, toss the sweet potato fries with olive oil, garlic powder, paprika, onion powder, smoked paprika, salt, and black pepper until evenly coated.
3. Spread the seasoned sweet potato fries in a single layer on the prepared baking sheet, making sure they are not overcrowded.
4. Bake in the preheated oven for 20-25 minutes, flipping halfway through, until the fries are golden brown and crispy.
5. Remove from the oven and let cool slightly before serving.
6. Serve the baked sweet potato fries hot with your favorite dipping sauce.

Nutritional Information (per serving):

- Calories: 180
- Protein: 2g
- Total Fats: 7g
- Fiber: 4g
- Carbohydrates: 28g

Spicy Hummus with Veggie Sticks

Time to Prepare: 10 minutes
Cooking Time: 0 minutes
Number of Servings: 6

Ingredients:

- 2 cans (15 ounces each) chickpeas, drained and rinsed
- 1/4 cup of tahini

- 1/4 cup of lemon juice
- 2 cloves garlic, minced
- 2 tablespoons olive oil
- 1 teaspoon of ground cumin
- 1/2 teaspoon of smoked paprika
- 1/4 teaspoon of cayenne pepper
- Salt to taste
- Assorted vegetable sticks (carrots, celery, cucumber, bell peppers) for serving

Instructions List:

1. In a food processor, combine the chickpeas, tahini, lemon juice, minced garlic, olive oil, ground cumin, smoked paprika, cayenne pepper, and a pinch of salt.
2. Blend until smooth and creamy, scraping down the sides of the bowl as needed. If the hummus is too thick, you can add a tablespoon of water at a time until desired consistency is reached.
3. Taste and adjust seasoning, adding more salt or lemon juice if needed.
4. Transfer the spicy hummus to a serving bowl and garnish with a drizzle of olive oil, a sprinkle of smoked paprika, and fresh herbs if desired.
5. Serve with assorted vegetable sticks for dipping.

Nutritional Information (per serving):

- Calories: 180
- Protein: 6g
- Total Fats: 9g
- Fiber: 6g
- Carbohydrates: 20g

Avocado Hummus

Time to Prepare: 10 minutes
Cooking Time: 0 minutes
Number of Servings: 6

Ingredients:

- 2 ripe avocados
- 1 can (15 ounces) chickpeas, drained and rinsed
- 1/4 cup of tahini
- 1/4 cup of fresh lemon juice
- 2 cloves garlic, minced
- 2 tablespoons olive oil

- 1/2 teaspoon of ground cumin
- Salt to taste
- Optional toppings: chopped cilantro, red pepper flakes

Instructions List:

1. Cut the avocados in half, remove the pits, and scoop the flesh into a food processor.
2. Add the drained chickpeas, tahini, lemon juice, minced garlic, olive oil, ground cumin, and a pinch of salt to the food processor.
3. Blend until smooth and creamy, scraping down the sides of the bowl as needed.
4. Taste and adjust seasoning, adding more salt or lemon juice if needed.
5. Transfer the avocado hummus to a serving bowl and garnish with optional toppings like chopped cilantro or red pepper flakes.
6. Serve with vegetable sticks, crackers, or pita bread.

Nutritional Information (per serving):

- Calories: 180
- Protein: 5g
- Total Fats: 11g
- Fiber: 7g
- Carbohydrates: 17g

Kale Chips with Nutritional Yeast

Time to Prepare: 10 minutes
Cooking Time: 15 minutes
Number of Servings: 4

Ingredients:

- 1 bunch kale, stems removed and leaves torn into bite-sized pieces
- 2 tablespoons olive oil
- 2 tablespoons nutritional yeast
- 1/2 teaspoon of garlic powder
- 1/2 teaspoon of onion powder
- Salt to taste

Instructions List:

1. Preheat the oven to 350°F (175°C) and line a baking sheet with parchment paper.
2. In a large bowl, toss the kale leaves with olive oil until evenly coated.
3. Sprinkle nutritional yeast, garlic powder, onion powder, and salt over the kale, and toss again to coat.
4. Spread the kale out in a single layer on the prepared baking sheet.

5. Bake in the preheated oven for 12-15 minutes, or until the kale is crispy but not burnt, checking and stirring halfway through.
   6. Remove from the oven and let cool slightly before serving.

Nutritional Information (per serving):

- Calories: 100
- Protein: 3g
- Total Fats: 7g
- Fiber: 2g
- Carbohydrates: 8g

Stuffed Mini Peppers with Quinoa

Time to Prepare: 20 minutes
Cooking Time: 25 minutes
Number of Servings: 6

Ingredients:

- 12 mini bell peppers, halved and seeds removed
- 1 cup of cooked quinoa
- 1 can (15 ounces) black beans, drained and rinsed
- 1 cup of corn kernels (fresh or frozen)
- 1 small onion, finely chopped
- 2 cloves garlic, minced
- 1 teaspoon of ground cumin
- 1 teaspoon of smoked paprika
- Salt and pepper to taste
- 1/4 cup of chopped fresh cilantro
- Juice of 1 lime
- Avocado slices, for serving (optional)

Instructions List:

1. Preheat the oven to 375°F (190°C) and line a baking sheet with parchment paper.
2. In a large bowl, combine cooked quinoa, black beans, corn, onion, garlic, cumin, smoked paprika, salt, pepper, cilantro, and lime juice. Mix well.
3. Stuff each halved mini pepper with the quinoa mixture and place them on the prepared baking sheet.
4. Bake in the preheated oven for 20-25 minutes, or until the peppers are tender.
5. Serve hot, optionally topped with avocado slices.

Nutritional Information (per serving):

- Calories: 180
- Protein: 7g
- Total Fats: 2g
- Fiber: 6g
- Carbohydrates: 35g

Garlic and Herb Roasted Nuts

Time to Prepare: 10 minutes
Cooking Time: 15 minutes
Number of Servings: 8

Ingredients:

- 2 cups of mixed raw nuts (almonds, cashews, walnuts, pecans)
- 2 tablespoons olive oil
- 2 cloves garlic, minced
- 1 teaspoon of dried thyme
- 1 teaspoon of dried rosemary
- 1/2 teaspoon of paprika
- Salt and pepper to taste

Instructions List:

1. Preheat the oven to 350°F (175°C) and line a baking sheet with parchment paper.
2. In a large bowl, combine the mixed nuts, olive oil, minced garlic, dried thyme, dried rosemary, paprika, salt, and pepper. Toss until the nuts are evenly coated.
3. Spread the seasoned nuts in a single layer on the prepared baking sheet.
4. Roast in the preheated oven for 12-15 minutes, stirring halfway through, until the nuts are golden and fragrant.
5. Remove from the oven and let cool completely before serving or storing in an airtight container.

Nutritional Information (per serving):

- Calories: 210
- Protein: 6g
- Total Fats: 18g
- Fiber: 3g
- Carbohydrates: 8g

Cucumber Avocado Rolls

Time to Prepare: 15 minutes
Cooking Time: 0 minutes
Number of Servings: 4

Ingredients:

- 2 large cucumbers
- 1 ripe avocado
- 1/4 cup of shredded carrots
- 1/4 cup of thinly sliced red bell pepper
- 1/4 cup of alfalfa sprouts
- 2 tablespoons chopped fresh cilantro
- 1 tablespoon lime juice
- Salt and pepper to taste
- Sesame seeds for garnish (optional)

Instructions List:

1. Slice the cucumbers lengthwise into thin strips using a vegetable peeler or mandoline slicer. Place the cucumber slices on a clean kitchen towel to absorb excess moisture.
2. In a small bowl, mash the ripe avocado with a fork. Stir in the shredded carrots, sliced red bell pepper, alfalfa sprouts, chopped cilantro, and lime juice. Season with salt and pepper to taste.
3. Lay a cucumber slice flat on a cutting board. Spoon a small amount of the avocado mixture onto one end of the cucumber slice.
4. Carefully roll the cucumber slice around the filling, forming a tight roll. Repeat with the remaining cucumber slices and filling.
5. Secure the rolls with toothpicks if needed. Sprinkle with sesame seeds for garnish if desired.
6. Serve immediately, or refrigerate until ready to serve.

Nutritional Information (per serving):

- Calories: 90
- Protein: 2g
- Total Fats: 7g
- Fiber: 4g
- Carbohydrates: 7g

Beetroot Hummus

Time to Prepare: 10 minutes
Cooking Time: 45 minutes (for roasting beetroots)
Number of Servings: 6

Ingredients:

- 2 medium-sized beetroots, roasted and peeled
- 1 can (15 oz) chickpeas, drained and rinsed
- 2 cloves garlic, minced
- 3 tablespoons tahini
- 2 tablespoons lemon juice
- 2 tablespoons extra virgin olive oil
- 1 teaspoon of ground cumin
- Salt and pepper to taste
- Water (as needed for consistency)

Instructions List:

1. Preheat the oven to 400°F (200°C). Wrap the beetroots individually in foil and roast them for about 45 minutes or until tender. Let them cool, then peel and roughly chop them.
2. In a food processor, combine the roasted beetroots, chickpeas, minced garlic, tahini, lemon juice, olive oil, ground cumin, salt, and pepper.
3. Blend until smooth, scraping down the sides of the processor as needed. If the mixture is too thick, add water, 1 tablespoon at a time, until desired consistency is reached.
4. Taste and adjust seasoning if necessary.
5. Transfer the beetroot hummus to a serving bowl. Drizzle with a little extra olive oil and garnish with sesame seeds, fresh herbs, or a sprinkle of paprika if desired.
6. Serve with vegetable sticks, pita bread, or crackers.

Nutritional Information (per serving):

- Calories: 120
- Protein: 4g
- Total Fats: 7g
- Fiber: 4g
- Carbohydrates: 12g

Turmeric Roasted Cauliflower

Time to Prepare: 10 minutes
Cooking Time: 25 minutes
Number of Servings: 4

Ingredients:

- 1 head cauliflower, cut into florets
- 2 tablespoons olive oil
- 1 teaspoon of ground turmeric

- 1/2 teaspoon of ground cumin
- 1/2 teaspoon of smoked paprika
- Salt and pepper to taste
- Fresh parsley or cilantro for garnish (optional)

Instructions List:

1. Preheat the oven to 425°F (220°C) and line a baking sheet with parchment paper.
2. In a large bowl, toss the cauliflower florets with olive oil, ground turmeric, ground cumin, smoked paprika, salt, and pepper until evenly coated.
3. Spread the cauliflower in a single layer on the prepared baking sheet.
4. Roast in the preheated oven for 20-25 minutes, or until the cauliflower is tender and golden brown, stirring halfway through.
5. Once roasted, remove from the oven and transfer to a serving dish.
6. Garnish with fresh parsley or cilantro if desired, and serve hot.

Nutritional Information (per serving):

- Calories: 90
- Protein: 3g
- Total Fats: 7g
- Fiber: 3g
- Carbohydrates: 7g

Carrot and Zucchini Fritters

Time to Prepare: 15 minutes
Cooking Time: 15 minutes
Number of Servings: 4

Ingredients:

- 2 medium carrots, grated
- 2 medium zucchinis, grated
- 1/2 cup of chickpea flour
- 2 tablespoons nutritional yeast
- 2 cloves garlic, minced
- 1 teaspoon of ground cumin
- 1/2 teaspoon of ground turmeric
- Salt and pepper to taste
- 2 tablespoons olive oil, for frying

Instructions List:

1. In a large mixing bowl, combine the grated carrots, grated zucchinis, chickpea flour, nutritional yeast, minced garlic, ground cumin, ground turmeric, salt, and pepper. Mix until well mixed.
2. Heat olive oil in a large skillet over medium heat.
3. Scoop about 1/4 cup of the fritter mixture and form into patties.
4. Place the patties in the skillet and cook for 3-4 minutes on each side, or until golden brown and crispy.
5. Once cooked, transfer the fritters to a plate lined with paper towels to drain excess oil.
6. Serve the fritters warm with your favorite dipping sauce or toppings.

Nutritional Information (per serving):

- Calories: 140
- Protein: 5g
- Total Fats: 6g
- Fiber: 5g
- Carbohydrates: 17g

Stuffed Mushrooms with Spinach

Time to Prepare: 15 minutes
Cooking Time: 20 minutes
Number of Servings: 4

Ingredients:

- 16 large button mushrooms, stems removed and finely chopped
- 2 cups of fresh spinach, chopped
- 1 small onion, finely chopped
- 2 cloves garlic, minced
- 1/4 cup of breadcrumbs (made from whole grain bread)
- 1/4 cup of nutritional yeast
- 2 tablespoons olive oil
- 1 teaspoon of dried oregano
- Salt and pepper to taste
- Fresh parsley, for garnish

Instructions List:

1. Preheat the oven to 375°F (190°C). Lightly grease a baking dish with olive oil.
2. In a skillet, heat 1 tablespoon of olive oil over medium heat. Add the chopped mushroom stems, onion, and garlic. Sauté until the onions are soft and translucent, about 5 minutes.
3. Add the chopped spinach to the skillet and cook until wilted, about 3 minutes.

4. Remove the skillet from the heat and stir in the breadcrumbs, nutritional yeast, dried oregano, salt, and pepper.
5. Stuff each mushroom cap with the spinach mixture and place them in the prepared baking dish.
6. Drizzle the stuffed mushrooms with the remaining olive oil.
7. Bake in the preheated oven for 15-20 minutes, or until the mushrooms are tender and lightly browned.
8. Garnish with fresh parsley before serving.

Nutritional Information (per serving):

- Calories: 120
- Protein: 5g
- Total Fats: 6g
- Fiber: 4g
- Carbohydrates: 14g

Edamame with Sea Salt

Time to Prepare: 5 minutes
Cooking Time: 5 minutes
Number of Servings: 4

Ingredients:

- 2 cups of frozen edamame in pods
- Sea salt, to taste

Instructions List:

1. Bring a pot of water to a boil.
2. Add the frozen edamame pods to the boiling water and cook for about 5 minutes, or until they are tender.
3. Drain the edamame and transfer them to a serving bowl.
4. Sprinkle with sea salt to taste.
5. Serve warm as a nutritious snack or appetizer.

Nutritional Information (per serving):

- Calories: 110
- Protein: 9g
- Total Fats: 4g
- Fiber: 8g
- Carbohydrates: 11g

Marinated Artichoke Hearts

Time to Prepare: 10 minutes
Cooking Time: 0 minutes
Number of Servings: 4

Ingredients:

- 1 can (14 oz) artichoke hearts, drained and rinsed
- 2 tablespoons extra virgin olive oil
- 2 tablespoons balsamic vinegar
- 2 cloves garlic, minced
- 1 teaspoon of dried oregano
- 1/2 teaspoon of dried basil
- Salt and black pepper, to taste
- Optional: red pepper flakes, for a spicy kick

Instructions List:

1. In a mixing bowl, combine the olive oil, balsamic vinegar, minced garlic, dried oregano, dried basil, salt, and black pepper. If desired, add red pepper flakes for some heat.
2. Add the drained and rinsed artichoke hearts to the bowl.
3. Toss the artichoke hearts gently until they are well coated with the marinade.
4. Cover the bowl and let the artichoke hearts marinate in the refrigerator for at least 1 hour, or preferably overnight, to allow the flavors to meld.
5. Serve chilled as a delicious appetizer or add them to salads, pasta dishes, or sandwiches for extra flavor.

Nutritional Information (per serving):

- Calories: 90
- Protein: 2g
- Total Fats: 7g
- Fiber: 3g
- Carbohydrates: 6g

Vegan Cheese Platter

Time to Prepare: 15 minutes
Cooking Time: 0 minutes
Number of Servings: 4

Ingredients:

- 1 cup of raw cashews, soaked for at least 4 hours
- 2 tablespoons nutritional yeast
- 2 tablespoons lemon juice

- 1 clove garlic, minced
- 1/2 teaspoon of onion powder
- 1/2 teaspoon of sea salt
- 2-3 tablespoons water, as needed
- Assorted crackers, sliced baguette, or vegetable sticks
- Fresh fruits, such as grapes or apple slices, for garnish
- Nuts and dried fruits, for variety

Instructions List:

1. Drain the soaked cashews and rinse them under cold water.
2. In a food processor or high-speed blender, combine the drained cashews, nutritional yeast, lemon juice, minced garlic, onion powder, and sea salt.
3. Blend the mixture until smooth and creamy, adding water gradually as needed to achieve the desired consistency.
4. Once the vegan cheese is creamy and smooth, transfer it to a serving bowl or plate.
5. Arrange the vegan cheese on a platter alongside assorted crackers, sliced baguette, or vegetable sticks.
6. Garnish the platter with fresh fruits, nuts, and dried fruits for variety.
7. Serve the vegan cheese platter as an appetizer or snack, and enjoy!

Nutritional Information (per serving):

- Calories: 220
- Protein: 7g
- Total Fats: 15g
- Fiber: 3g
- Carbohydrates: 16g

Chapter 7: Desserts

Dark Chocolate Avocado Mousse

Time to Prepare: 10 minutes
Cooking Time: 0 minutes
Number of Servings: 4

Ingredients:

- 2 ripe avocados
- 1/4 cup of cocoa powder
- 1/4 cup of maple syrup or agave nectar
- 1 teaspoon of vanilla extract
- Pinch of sea salt
- Fresh berries, for garnish (optional)

Instructions List:

1. Cut the avocados in half, remove the pits, and scoop the flesh into a blender or food processor.
2. Add the cocoa powder, maple syrup or agave nectar, vanilla extract, and a pinch of sea salt to the blender.
3. Blend the ingredients until smooth and creamy, scraping down the sides of the blender or food processor as needed.
4. Once the mixture is smooth, transfer it to serving dishes or ramekins.
5. Chill the mousse in the refrigerator for at least 30 minutes before serving.
6. Garnish with fresh berries, if desired, and serve chilled.

Nutritional Information (per serving):

- Calories: 210
- Protein: 3g
- Total Fats: 15g
- Fiber: 7g
- Carbohydrates: 20g

Coconut Chia Pudding

Time to Prepare: 5 minutes
Cooking Time: 0 minutes
Number of Servings: 4

Ingredients:

- 1/2 cup of chia seeds
- 2 cups of coconut milk (unsweetened)

- 2 tablespoons maple syrup or agave nectar
- 1 teaspoon of vanilla extract
- Fresh berries, for topping (optional)
- Shredded coconut, for topping (optional)

Instructions List:

1. In a mixing bowl, combine the chia seeds, coconut milk, maple syrup or agave nectar, and vanilla extract.
2. Whisk the ingredients together until well mixed.
3. Cover the bowl and refrigerate for at least 2 hours, or preferably overnight, to allow the chia seeds to absorb the liquid and thicken.
4. Once the pudding has thickened to your desired consistency, stir well.
5. Divide the pudding into serving dishes or jars.
6. Top with fresh berries and shredded coconut, if desired, before serving.

Nutritional Information (per serving):

- Calories: 220
- Protein: 5g
- Total Fats: 15g
- Fiber: 10g
- Carbohydrates: 20g

Almond Butter Cookies

Time to Prepare: 10 minutes
Cooking Time: 10 minutes
Number of Servings: 12 cookies

Ingredients:

- 1 cup of almond butter
- 1/2 cup of coconut sugar
- 1 flax egg (1 tablespoon ground flaxseed meal + 3 tablespoons water)
- 1 teaspoon of vanilla extract
- 1/2 teaspoon of baking soda
- Pinch of salt

Instructions List:

1. Preheat your oven to 350°F (175°C) and line a baking sheet with parchment paper.
2. In a large mixing bowl, prepare the flax egg by mixing together the ground flaxseed meal and water. Let it sit for a few minutes to thicken.

3. Add the almond butter, coconut sugar, vanilla extract, baking soda, and salt to the bowl with the flax egg. Mix until well mixed.

4. Scoop out tablespoon-sized portions of dough and roll them into balls. Place them on the prepared baking sheet, leaving some space between each cookie.

5. Use a fork to gently flatten each cookie, creating a crisscross pattern on top.

6. Bake in the preheated oven for 8-10 minutes, or until the edges are golden brown.

7. Remove from the oven and let the cookies cool on the baking sheet for a few minutes before transferring them to a wire rack to cool completely.

Nutritional Information (per serving - 1 cookie):

- Calories: 150
- Protein: 4g
- Total Fats: 10g
- Fiber: 2g
- Carbohydrates: 12g

Baked Cinnamon Apples

Time to Prepare: 10 minutes
Cooking Time: 25 minutes
Number of Servings: 4 servings

Ingredients:

- 4 medium apples, cored and sliced
- 2 tablespoons maple syrup
- 1 tablespoon lemon juice
- 1 teaspoon of ground cinnamon
- Pinch of nutmeg
- Pinch of salt

Instructions List:

1. Preheat your oven to 375°F (190°C) and lightly grease a baking dish.

2. In a large bowl, combine the sliced apples, maple syrup, lemon juice, cinnamon, nutmeg, and salt. Toss until the apples are evenly coated.

3. Transfer the coated apples to the prepared baking dish, spreading them out into an even layer.

4. Bake in the preheated oven for 20-25 minutes, or until the apples are tender and caramelized, stirring halfway through.

5. Remove from the oven and let cool slightly before serving.

Nutritional Information (per serving):

- Calories: 120

- Protein: 0g
- Total Fats: 0g
- Fiber: 4g
- Carbohydrates: 32g

Berry Chia Parfait

Time to Prepare: 10 minutes
Cooking Time: 0 minutes
Number of Servings: 2 servings

Ingredients:

- 1 cup of mixed berries (such as strawberries, blueberries, raspberries)
- 2 tablespoons chia seeds
- 1 cup of plant-based yogurt
- 1 tablespoon maple syrup (optional)
- 1/4 teaspoon of vanilla extract
- 2 tablespoons granola (optional, for topping)

Instructions List:

1. In a bowl, mash half of the mixed berries with a fork to release their juices.
2. Stir in the chia seeds, plant-based yogurt, maple syrup (if using), and vanilla extract. Mix well to combine.
3. Cover the bowl and refrigerate for at least 2 hours, or overnight, to allow the chia seeds to thicken.
4. To assemble the parfaits, divide the chia mixture evenly between two serving glasses or bowls.
5. Top each parfait with the remaining mixed berries and granola, if desired.
6. Serve immediately and enjoy!

Nutritional Information (per serving):

- Calories: 180
- Protein: 5g
- Total Fats: 6g
- Fiber: 10g
- Carbohydrates: 25g

Mango Sorbet

Time to Prepare: 10 minutes
Cooking Time: 0 minutes
Number of Servings: 4 servings

Ingredients:

- 3 cups of frozen mango chunks
- 1/4 cup of plant-based milk (such as almond milk or coconut milk)
- 2 tablespoons maple syrup (optional, adjust to taste)
- 1 tablespoon lime juice

Instructions List:

1. Place the frozen mango chunks, plant-based milk, maple syrup (if using), and lime juice in a blender or food processor.
2. Blend until smooth and creamy, scraping down the sides of the blender or food processor as needed.
3. If the mixture is too thick, add more plant-based milk, a tablespoon at a time, until desired consistency is reached.
4. Once smooth, transfer the sorbet mixture to a freezer-safe container.
5. Freeze for at least 2 hours, or until firm.
6. Before serving, let the sorbet sit at room temperature for a few minutes to soften slightly.
7. Scoop the mango sorbet into bowls or cones, and enjoy!

Nutritional Information (per serving):

- Calories: 110
- Protein: 1g
- Total Fats: 1g
- Fiber: 3g
- Carbohydrates: 27g

Matcha Green Tea Ice Cream

Time to Prepare: 10 minutes
Cooking Time: 4 hours (chilling time)
Number of Servings: 4 servings

Ingredients:

- 2 cans (13.5 oz each) full-fat coconut milk, chilled in the refrigerator overnight
- 1/2 cup of maple syrup or agave nectar
- 2 tablespoons matcha green tea powder
- 1 teaspoon of vanilla extract
- Pinch of salt

Instructions List:

1. Begin by chilling a large mixing bowl in the freezer for about 10 minutes.
2. Open the chilled cans of coconut milk without shaking them. Scoop out the thick coconut cream that has risen to the top and place it in the chilled mixing bowl. Reserve the coconut water for another use.

3. Using a hand mixer or stand mixer, beat the coconut cream on high speed until fluffy and smooth, about 2-3 minutes.

4. Add the maple syrup or agave nectar, matcha green tea powder, vanilla extract, and a pinch of salt to the whipped coconut cream.

5. Continue to beat on high speed until all ingredients are well mixed and the mixture is smooth and creamy.

6. Transfer the mixture to a freezer-safe container, cover, and freeze for at least 4 hours, or until firm.

7. Before serving, let the ice cream sit at room temperature for a few minutes to soften slightly.

8. Scoop the matcha green tea ice cream into bowls or cones, and enjoy!

Nutritional Information (per serving):

- Calories: 360
- Protein: 3g
- Total Fats: 29g
- Fiber: 1g
- Carbohydrates: 28g

Vegan Lemon Bars

Time to Prepare: 15 minutes
Cooking Time: 35 minutes
Number of Servings: 12 bars

Ingredients:

- For the crust:
    - 1 cup of almond flour
    - 1/4 cup of coconut oil, melted
    - 2 tablespoons maple syrup
    - Pinch of salt
- For the filling:
    - 1 cup of raw cashews, soaked in water for 4 hours or overnight, then drained
    - 1/2 cup of full-fat coconut milk
    - 1/3 cup lemon juice
    - 1/4 cup of maple syrup
    - 2 tablespoons arrowroot powder
    - Zest of 1 lemon
    - Pinch of turmeric (for color, optional)

Instructions List:

1. Preheat your oven to 350°F (175°C). Line an 8x8-inch baking dish with parchment paper, leaving some overhang for easy removal.
2. In a mixing bowl, combine the almond flour, melted coconut oil, maple syrup, and a pinch of salt for the crust. Mix until well mixed and crumbly.
3. Press the crust mixture evenly into the bottom of the prepared baking dish. Bake in the preheated oven for 10-12 minutes, or until lightly golden brown. Remove from the oven and set aside.
4. In a blender, combine the soaked cashews, coconut milk, lemon juice, maple syrup, arrowroot powder, lemon zest, and turmeric (if using) for the filling. Blend until smooth and creamy.
5. Pour the filling mixture over the baked crust and spread it out evenly.
6. Return the baking dish to the oven and bake for another 20-25 minutes, or until the filling is set.
7. Once baked, remove from the oven and let it cool to room temperature. Then transfer to the refrigerator to chill for at least 2 hours, or until firm.
8. Once chilled, use the parchment paper overhang to lift the lemon bars out of the baking dish. Cut into squares or bars.
9. Serve chilled and enjoy!

Nutritional Information (per serving):

- Calories: 210
- Protein: 4g
- Total Fats: 16g
- Fiber: 2g
- Carbohydrates: 14g

Chocolate-Dipped Strawberries

Time to Prepare: 15 minutes
Cooking Time: 5 minutes
Number of Servings: 4 servings

Ingredients:

- 1 cup of vegan dark chocolate chips
- 1 tablespoon coconut oil
- 1 pint fresh strawberries, washed and dried

Instructions List:

1. In a microwave-safe bowl, combine the vegan dark chocolate chips and coconut oil. Microwave in 30-second intervals, stirring in between, until the chocolate is fully melted and smooth.
2. Holding each strawberry by the stem, dip it into the melted chocolate, swirling to coat about two-thirds of the berry.
3. Allow any excess chocolate to drip off, then place the dipped strawberry on a parchment-lined baking sheet.
4. Repeat the dipping process with the remaining strawberries.

5. Once all the strawberries are dipped, transfer the baking sheet to the refrigerator to allow the chocolate to set for about 30 minutes.

6. Once the chocolate has set, remove the strawberries from the refrigerator and serve immediately, or store them in an airtight container in the refrigerator for up to 3 days.

Nutritional Information (per serving):

- Calories: 180
- Protein: 2g
- Total Fats: 11g
- Fiber: 5g
- Carbohydrates: 22g

Raw Brownie Bites

Time to Prepare: 15 minutes
Cooking Time: 0 minutes
Number of Servings: 12 servings

Ingredients:

- 1 cup of Medjool dates, pitted
- 1 cup of walnuts
- 2 tablespoons cocoa powder
- Pinch of sea salt
- 1/2 teaspoon of vanilla extract
- 2 tablespoons almond butter
- 2 tablespoons shredded coconut (optional, for coating)

Instructions List:

1. In a food processor, combine the pitted Medjool dates, walnuts, cocoa powder, sea salt, vanilla extract, and almond butter.
2. Pulse the ingredients until they are well mixed and form a sticky dough.
3. Scoop out about 1 tablespoon of the dough at a time and roll it into balls.
4. If desired, roll the balls in shredded coconut to coat.
5. Place the brownie bites in an airtight container and store them in the refrigerator for at least 30 minutes to firm up before serving.

Nutritional Information (per serving):

- Calories: 120
- Protein: 2g
- Total Fats: 7g
- Fiber: 3g

- Carbohydrates: 14g

Pineapple Coconut Smoothie Bowl

Time to Prepare: 10 minutes
Cooking Time: 0 minutes
Number of Servings: 2 servings

Ingredients:

- 2 cups of frozen pineapple chunks
- 1 ripe banana
- 1/2 cup of coconut milk
- 1/4 cup of rolled oats
- 1 tablespoon chia seeds
- 1 tablespoon shredded coconut (plus more for topping)
- Sliced fresh fruit (such as berries or kiwi), for topping
- Granola, for topping (optional)

Instructions List:

1. In a blender, combine the frozen pineapple chunks, ripe banana, coconut milk, rolled oats, chia seeds, and shredded coconut.
2. Blend on high until smooth and creamy, adding more coconut milk if needed to reach your desired consistency.
3. Pour the smoothie mixture into bowls.
4. Top with sliced fresh fruit, additional shredded coconut, and granola if desired.
5. Serve immediately and enjoy!

Nutritional Information (per serving):

- Calories: 275
- Protein: 4g
- Total Fats: 13g
- Fiber: 8g
- Carbohydrates: 41g

Pumpkin Pie Bites

Time to Prepare: 15 minutes
Cooking Time: 25 minutes
Number of Servings: 12 servings

Ingredients:

- 1 cup of rolled oats

- 1/2 cup of almond flour
- 1/4 cup of maple syrup
- 1/4 cup of coconut oil, melted
- 1 cup of pumpkin puree
- 2 tablespoons ground flaxseed
- 1 teaspoon of vanilla extract
- 1 teaspoon of ground cinnamon
- 1/2 teaspoon of ground ginger
- 1/4 teaspoon of ground nutmeg
- 1/4 teaspoon of ground cloves
- Pinch of salt

Instructions List:

1. Preheat the oven to 350°F (175°C). Grease a mini muffin tin with coconut oil or line it with paper liners.
2. In a large bowl, combine the rolled oats, almond flour, maple syrup, and melted coconut oil. Mix well until the mixture forms a dough.
3. Press the dough evenly into the bottom and up the sides of each mini muffin cup to form crusts.
4. In another bowl, mix together the pumpkin puree, ground flaxseed, vanilla extract, ground cinnamon, ground ginger, ground nutmeg, ground cloves, and a pinch of salt until well mixed.
5. Spoon the pumpkin mixture into each crust, filling each nearly to the top.
6. Bake in the preheated oven for 25 minutes, or until the crust is golden brown and the filling is set.
7. Remove from the oven and let cool in the muffin tin for 10 minutes before transferring the pumpkin pie bites to a wire rack to cool completely.
8. Once cooled, serve and enjoy!

Nutritional Information (per serving):

- Calories: 123
- Protein: 2g
- Total Fats: 7g
- Fiber: 2g
- Carbohydrates: 13g

30-DAY MEAL PLAN

Day	Breakfast	Lunch	Dinner
1	Blueberry Chia Pudding	Kale and Avocado Salad	Chickpea and Spinach Patties
2	Sweet Potato and Black Bean Breakfast Tacos	Curried Lentil Soup	Turmeric Cauliflower Rice Salad
3	Quinoa Breakfast Bowl	Roasted Tomato Basil Soup	BBQ Jackfruit Sandwiches
4	Turmeric Spiced Oatmeal	Miso Soup with Tofu and Greens	Vegan Meatloaf with Lentils and Walnuts
5	Avocado Toast with Pomegranate Seeds	Sweet Potato and Carrot Soup	Seitan Stir-Fry with Vegetables
6	Spinach and Mushroom Breakfast Scramble	Broccoli and Kale Soup	Tempeh Tacos with Avocado
7	Almond Butter Banana Smoothie Bowl	Coconut Curry Butternut Squash Soup	Portobello Mushroom Steaks
8	Vegan Breakfast Burrito	Spiced Chickpea and Spinach Stew	Chickpea and Quinoa Stuffed Peppers
9	Cinnamon Apple Overnight Oats	Cauliflower Leek Soup	Vegan Shepherd's Pie
10	Green Detox Smoothie	Tomato and Red Pepper Soup	Grilled Tofu with Chimichurri Sauce
11	Sweet Potato and Kale Hash	Zucchini and Basil Soup	Eggplant Rollatini with Cashew Ricotta
12	Vegan French Toast	Mushroom and Barley Soup	Spicy Lentil and Vegetable Stew
13	Chia Seed Strawberry Parfait	Gingered Carrot Soup	Pulled Jackfruit Tacos
14	Pumpkin Spice Muffins	Sweet Corn and Quinoa Soup	Vegan Tuna Salad with Chickpeas
15	Spelt Flour Pancakes	Red Lentil and Spinach Soup	Watermelon Poke Bowl
16	Turmeric Ginger Tea	Kale and Avocado Salad	Chickpea and Spinach Patties
17	Green Tea Matcha Latte	Rainbow Quinoa Salad	Black Bean and Sweet Potato Burgers
18	Berry Beet Smoothie	Spinach and Strawberry Salad	BBQ Jackfruit Sandwiches
19	Golden Milk Latte	Roasted Beet and Orange Salad	Vegan Meatloaf with Lentils and Walnuts
20	Pineapple Ginger Smoothie	Cucumber and Tomato Salad with Mint	Seitan Stir-Fry with Vegetables
21	Mint Cucumber Detox Water	Arugula and Pear Salad	Tempeh Tacos with Avocado
22	Anti-Inflammatory Green Juice	Warm Lentil and Sweet Potato Salad	Portobello Mushroom Steaks
23	Spiced Apple Cider	Broccoli and Cranberry Salad	Chickpea and Quinoa Stuffed Peppers
24	Mango Turmeric Smoothie	Turmeric Cauliflower Rice Salad	Vegan Shepherd's Pie
25	Hibiscus Iced Tea	Asian Sesame Cabbage Salad	Grilled Tofu with Chimichurri Sauce
26	Lemon Ginger Infused Water	Grilled Vegetable Salad	Eggplant Rollatini with Cashew Ricotta
27	Pomegranate Green Tea	Mediterranean Farro Salad	Spicy Lentil and Vegetable Stew
28	Cherry Basil Lemonade	Mango Black Bean Salad	Pulled Jackfruit Tacos

| 29 | Carrot Orange Ginger Juice | Spicy Thai Peanut Noodle Salad | Vegan Tuna Salad with Chickpeas |
| 30 | Blueberry Basil Smoothie | Chia Seed Strawberry Parfait | Watermelon Poke Bow |

MEASUREMENT CONVERSION TABLE

Measurement	Imperial (US)	Metric
Volume		
1 teaspoon of	1 tsp	5 milliliters
1 tablespoon	1 tbsp	15 milliliters
1 fluid ounce	1 fl oz	30 milliliters
1 cup of	1 cup of	240 milliliters
1 pint	1 pt	473 milliliters
1 quart	1 qt	0.95 liters
1 gallon	1 gal	3.8 liters
Weight		
1 ounce	1 oz	28 grams
1 pound	1 lb	454 grams
Temperature		
32°F	32°F	0°C
212°F	212°F	100°C
Other		
1 stick of butter	1 stick	113 grams

CONCLUSION

Our cookbook features a wide range of delicious plant-based recipes that are incredibly flavorful and good for your body. These recipes provide a tasty way to promote overall health and well-being by using whole, nutrient-rich ingredients and incorporating anti-inflammatory spices and herbs.

Our menu offers a wide range of delicious breakfast options, including Blueberry Chia Pudding and Sweet Potato and Black Bean Breakfast Tacos. For those looking for a more filling meal, we have BBQ Jackfruit Sandwiches and Vegan Shepherd's Pie. Each recipe is carefully designed to provide both great taste and nutritional value. Our menu includes a wide variety of soups, salads, snacks, and desserts to cater to all your plant-based meal needs. Whether you're looking for a light snack or a hearty meal, we've got you covered.

We've made sure to feature beverages like Turmeric Ginger Tea and Pineapple Ginger Smoothie, emphasizing the significance of staying hydrated and the advantages of adding anti-inflammatory ingredients to your drinks.

Whether you're a beginner or an experienced plant-based eater, this cookbook has something for everyone who wants to enjoy a tasty and healthy diet. These recipes offer a delicious and nutritious culinary experience by utilizing the benefits of plant-based ingredients and focusing on reducing inflammation. Cheers to a life filled with good health and enjoyable meals!

RECIPES INDEX

Almond Butter Banana Smoothie Bowl 11

Almond Butter Cookies 88

Anti-Inflammatory Green Juice 24

Arugula and Pear Salad 49

Asian Sesame Cabbage Salad 52

Avocado Hummus 76

Avocado Toast with Pomegranate Seeds 9

Baked Cinnamon Apples 89

Baked Sweet Potato Fries 75

BBQ Jackfruit Sandwiches 60

Beetroot Hummus 80

Berry Beet Smoothie 20

Berry Chia Parfait 90

Black Bean and Sweet Potato Burgers 59

Blueberry Basil Smoothie 29

Blueberry Chia Pudding 6

Broccoli and Cranberry Salad 50

Broccoli and Kale Soup 34

Carrot and Zucchini Fritters 82

Carrot Orange Ginger Juice 28

Cauliflower Leek Soup 38

Cherry Basil Lemonade 27

Chia Seed Strawberry Parfait 15

Chickpea and Quinoa Stuffed Peppers 65

Chickpea and Spinach Patties 58

Chocolate-Dipped Strawberries 93

Cinnamon Apple Overnight Oats 12

Coconut Chia Pudding 87

Coconut Curry Butternut Squash Soup 36

Cucumber and Tomato Salad with Mint 48

Cucumber Avocado Rolls 80

Curried Lentil Soup 30

Dark Chocolate Avocado Mousse 87

Edamame with Sea Salt 84

Eggplant Rollatini with Cashew Ricotta 68

Garlic and Herb Roasted Nuts 79

Gingered Carrot Soup 41

Golden Milk Latte 21

Green Detox Smoothie 13

Green Tea Matcha Latte 19

Grilled Tofu with Chimichurri Sauce 67

Grilled Vegetable Salad 53

Hibiscus Iced Tea 25

Kale and Avocado Salad 45

Kale Chips with Nutritional Yeast 77

Lemon Ginger Infused Water 26

Mango Black Bean Salad 55

Mango Sorbet 90

Mango Turmeric Smoothie 25

Marinated Artichoke Hearts 84

Matcha Green Tea Ice Cream 91

Mediterranean Farro Salad 54

Mint Cucumber Detox Water 22

Miso Soup with Tofu and Greens 32

Mushroom and Barley Soup 40

Pineapple Coconut Smoothie Bowl 95

Pineapple Ginger Smoothie 21

Pomegranate Green Tea 27

Portobello Mushroom Steaks 64

Pulled Jackfruit Tacos 70

Pumpkin Pie Bites 95

Pumpkin Spice Muffins 16

Quinoa Breakfast Bowl 7

Rainbow Quinoa Salad 45

Raw Brownie Bites 94

Red Lentil and Spinach Soup 43

Roasted Beet and Orange Salad 47

Roasted Chickpeas 74

Roasted Tomato Basil Soup 31

Seitan Stir-Fry with Vegetables 62

Spelt Flour Pancakes 17

Spiced Apple Cider 23

Spiced Chickpea and Spinach Stew 37

Spicy Hummus with Veggie Sticks 75

Spicy Lentil and Vegetable Stew 69

Spicy Thai Peanut Noodle Salad 56

Spinach and Mushroom Breakfast Scramble 10

Spinach and Strawberry Salad 46

Stuffed Mini Peppers with Quinoa 78

Stuffed Mushrooms with Spinach 83

Sweet Corn and Quinoa Soup 42

Sweet Potato and Black Bean Breakfast Tacos 6

Sweet Potato and Carrot Soup 33

Sweet Potato and Kale Hash 14

Tempeh Tacos with Avocado 63

Tomato and Red Pepper Soup 39

Turmeric Cauliflower Rice Salad 51

Turmeric Ginger Tea 19

Turmeric Ginger Vegetable Soup 35

Turmeric Roasted Cauliflower 81

Turmeric Spiced Oatmeal 8

Vegan Breakfast Burrito 11

Vegan Cheese Platter 85

Vegan French Toast 15

Vegan Lemon Bars 92

Vegan Meatloaf with Lentils and Walnuts 61

Vegan Shepherd's Pie 66

Vegan Tuna Salad with Chickpeas 71

Warm Lentil and Sweet Potato Salad 49

Watermelon Poke Bowl 72

Zucchini and Basil Soup 39

Printed in Great Britain
by Amazon